Histoplasma and Histoplasmosis

Edited by Felix Bongomin

Published in London, United Kingdom

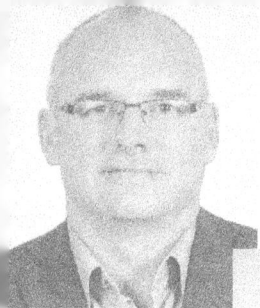
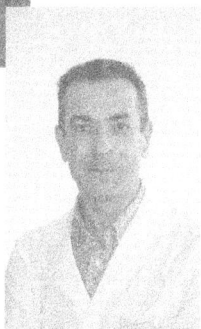
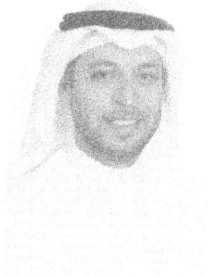
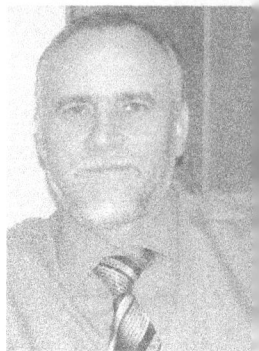
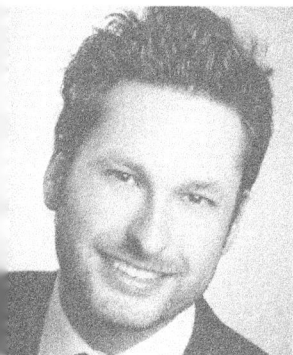
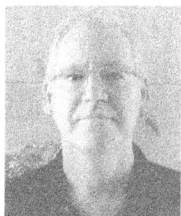
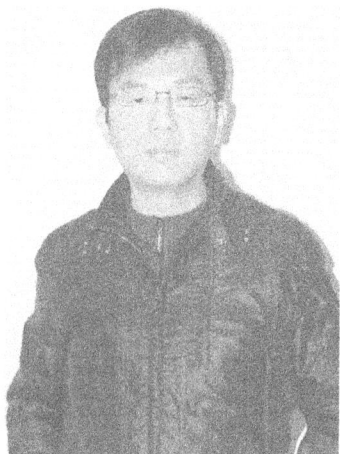

IntechOpen

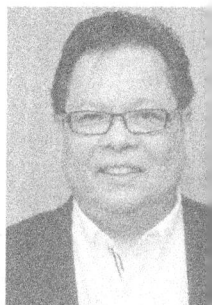
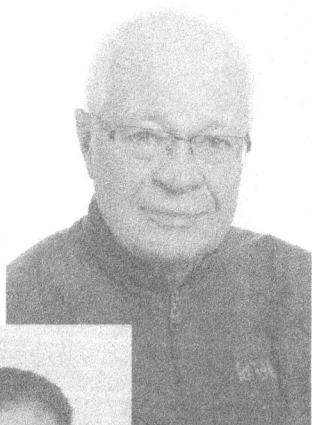
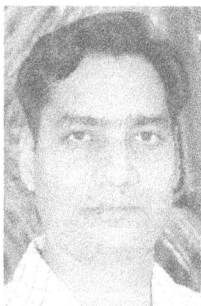
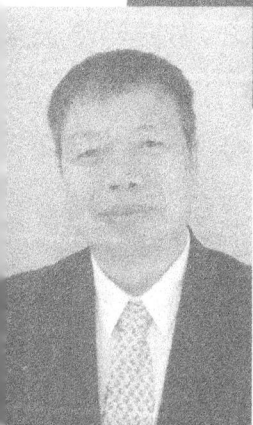
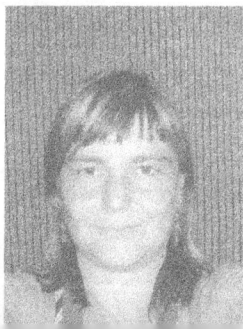
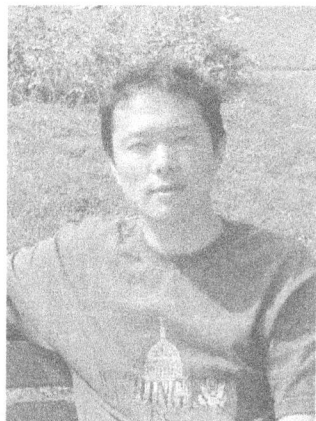

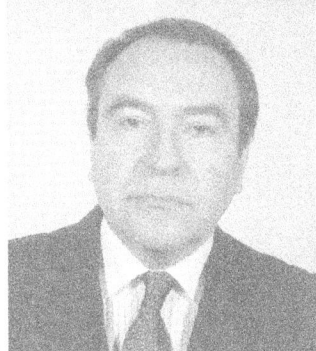

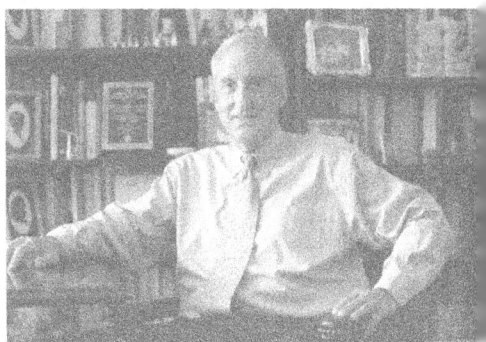

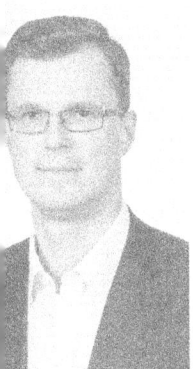

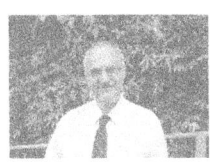

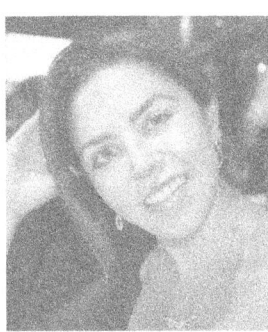

Supporting open minds since 2005

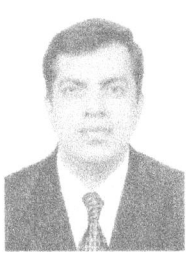

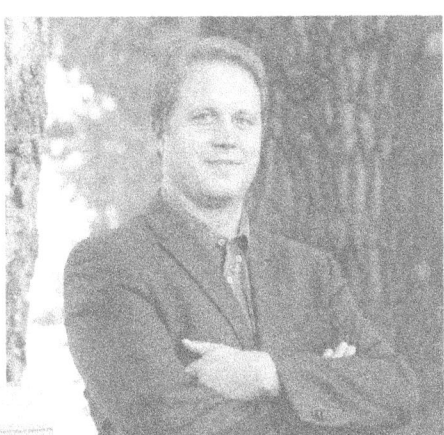

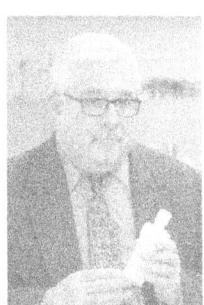

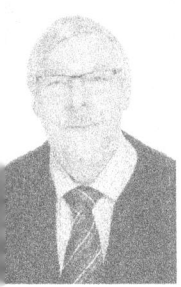

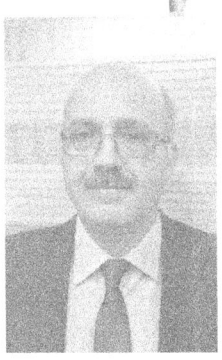

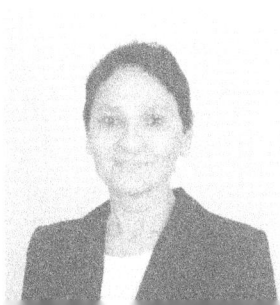

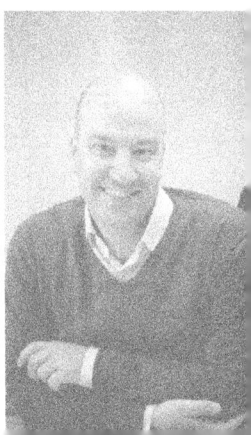

Histoplasma and Histoplasmosis
http://dx.doi.org/10.5772/intechopen.87271
Edited by Felix Bongomin

Contributors
Maria J Buitrago, Clara Valero, Findra Setianingrum, Anna Rozaliyani, Magalie Demar, Emilie Guemas, Loic Sobanska, Felix Bongomin, Richard Kwizera, Joseph Baluku, Lucy Grace Asio, Akaninyene Otu, Lauryn Nsenga

Notice
Statements and opinions expressed in the chapters are these of the individual contributors and not necessarily those of the editors or publisher. No responsibility is accepted for the accuracy of information contained in the published chapters. The publisher assumes no responsibility for any damage or injury to persons or property arising out of the use of any materials, instructions, methods or ideas contained in the book.

First published in London, United Kingdom, 2020 by IntechOpen
IntechOpen is the global imprint of INTECHOPEN LIMITED, registered in England and Wales, registration number: 11086078, 7th floor, 10 Lower Thames Street, London, EC3R 6AF, United Kingdom
Printed in Croatia

British Library Cataloguing-in-Publication Data
A catalogue record for this book is available from the British Library

Additional hard and PDF copies can be obtained from orders@intechopen.com

Histoplasma and Histoplasmosis
Edited by Felix Bongomin
p. cm.
Print ISBN 978-1-83962-961-7
Online ISBN 978-1-83962-962-4
eBook (PDF) ISBN 978-1-83962-963-1

We are IntechOpen,
the world's leading publisher of
Open Access books

Built by scientists, for scientists

5,000+
Open access books available

125,000+
International authors and editors

140M+
Downloads

Our authors are among the

151
Countries delivered to

Top 1%
most cited scientists

12.2%
Contributors from top 500 universities

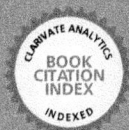

Interested in publishing with us?
Contact book.department@intechopen.com

Numbers displayed above are based on latest data collected.
For more information visit www.intechopen.com

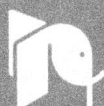

Meet the editor

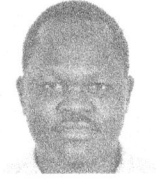

Dr. Felix Bongomin is an internationally recognised expert in clinical mycology and a resident internal medicine physician. His clinical and research interests are in histoplasmosis, aspergillosis, cryptococcosis, and fungal disease epidemiology. He is currently a lecturer in the Department of Medical Microbiology and Immunology, Gulu University School of Medicine, Gulu, Uganda. Dr. Bongomin is actively involved in the teaching of both medical and public health students in various aspects of medical microbiology and immunology. In the past five years, he has contributed to more than fifty international peer-reviewed articles and book chapters, with more than 600 citations.

Contents

Preface

"...only the prepared mind can help the impaired host.."

Dr. Libero Ajello

Histoplasma and Histoplasmosis is a book of general medical interest to undergraduate and postgraduate students and specialist healthcare practitioners in the field of clinical and laboratory practices. This book provides comprehensive yet "bite-sized" background knowledge and updates in the recent understanding of the histoplasma organism and the disease it causes to trainees and practicing mycologists at all degrees of experience.

This book was written through a collective and collaborative work of leading, internationally recognised authors in the field of infectious diseases, medical mycology, and microbiology and laboratory medicine. The editor judiciously curated individual chapter contributions into a single text to maintain the relevance and the scope of this book without compromising the science within it.

Histoplasma capsulatum var. capsulatum and *Histoplasma capsulatum var. duboisii* and the human disease they cause, collectively referred to as histoplasmosis, are prevalent worldwide, although certain areas are hyperendemic for this disease. The World Health Organization has officially recognised histoplasmosis as an AIDS-defining illness, a neglected tropical (fungal) disease, and an important cause of death in patients with advanced HIV disease. Histoplasmosis has an incredibly protean manifestation and is commonly misdiagnosed as tuberculosis or cancer. In the recent past, significant advancement has been achieved with respect to diagnostic and therapeutic approaches.

This book discusses the global distribution of the disease, provides an updated estimation of the burden of histoplasmosis in Asia, and examines recent advances in laboratory diagnosis and treatment of histoplasma and histoplasmosis.

I hope this book will pique interest in histoplasmosis and eventually save many lives from this devastating disease. I welcome constructive criticisms.

Dr. Felix Bongomin, MB ChB, MSc
School of Medicine,
Gulu University,
Gulu City, Uganda

Section 1

Introduction

Chapter 1

Introductory Chapter: The Global Distribution of Human Histoplasmosis - An Overview

Felix Bongomin and Lauryn Nsenga

1. Introduction

Between 1906 and 1909, Dr. Samuel T. Darling described human histoplasmosis (of Darling or Darling's disease) among three patients in the Canal Zone, Panama who had presented with severe emaciation, pancytopenia, intermittent fevers and splenomegaly – resembling kala-azar and disseminated tuberculosis, clinically [1]. Dr. Darling demonstrated numerous small, intracellular encapsulated micro-organisms in tissue specimens of his patients and named the organism, *Histoplasma capsulatum* [2].

H. capsulatum is a thermally dimorphic fungus, existing as a mould in the environment and as a small narrow-based budding yeast in the host at 37°C. Environmental isolations of the fungus have been made from soil enriched with excreta from chicken, starlings, and bats [3, 4]. *H. capsulatum* species complex comprises of two distinct varieties, that is, *H. capsulatum var. capsulatum* (hereafter referred to as *H. capsulatum*) and *H. capsulatum var. duboisii* (hereafter referred to as *H. duboisii*) [5]. Epidemiologically, *H. capsulatum* is patchily distributed around the world, whereas *H. duboisii* is almost restricted to Sub-Saharan Africa [6]. Histologically, the yeast form of *H. capsulatum* is smaller, about 1–5 μm compared to the larger *H. duboisii*, which is about 5–20 μm [7]. Clinically, *H. capsulatum* is associated with protean manifestations; meanwhile *H. duboisii* mainly causes musculoskeletal and cutaneous manifestations [8, 9]. Both species complex are associated with pulmonary diseases; however, the absence of pulmonary lesions does not exclude the diagnosis of other forms of histoplasmosis [8].

Humans acquire histoplasmosis through inhalation of *Histoplasma* microconidia (spores) from abiotic environment. Majority of the immunocompetent individuals are asymptomatic, some develop self-limiting influenza-like syndromes and a vast minority develop disseminated disease, especially those with severe immunosup-pression such as those with HIV/AIDS and those on biologic therapy [10, 11]. Subclinical infections can be demonstrated through histoplasmin skin testing while clinical disease through conventional culture and microscopy or histopathological analysis of the appropriate clinical specimen [12–14]. In this chapter, we aimed to overview the global epidemiology of histoplasmosis and also we touched briefly on its clinical manifestations, diagnosis, and treatment.

2. Global epidemiology

The global distribution of histoplasmosis and *Histoplasma* is incompletely understood [15]. The true burden of histoplasmosis in many areas of the world remains unknown due to lack of diagnostics, awareness among clinicians, and in histoplasmosis not being a notifiable disease. *Histoplasma* inhabits soils enriched with bird and bat excreta, high nitrogen content with a neutral PH [16]. Occupational exposures among excavators and those at construction sites resulting into disruption of soil and inhalation of large inoculum of *Histoplasma* spores have been described [17].

Despite the global report of histoplasmosis, majority of the cases are reported from North and Latin America [6, 15, 18]. In North America, the Ohio and Mississippi river valleys and the Atlantic coastal states of Florida and New York have high rates of prior sub-clinical histoplasmosis based on histoplasmin skin tests [6, 15, 18]. Histoplasmosis in South and Central America is heavily driven by the HIV pandemic, and AIDS-associated histoplasmosis remains as common as tuberculosis in this region [19–21]. Imported and autochthonous cases of histoplasmosis have been described in Europe. Likewise in Africa, microfoci of histoplasmosis exist with reported large and small outbreaks have been attributed to histoplasmosis, but most infections are sporadic and imported cases from endemic areas have also been described [15, 22]. In review of literature of recently published data, chronic cavitary histoplasmosis is described as a common entity in endemic areas and commonly misdiagnosed as smear-negative tuberculosis [23].

In HIV population, globally, about half a million people get infected with *Histoplasma* infection every year. However, approximately 100,000 people develop disseminated disease [24, 25], with mortality rates if treated ranging between 30 to 50% and 100% if not [20, 21, 26–29]. Accordingly, WHO has recognised as a killer of patients with advanced HIV and has currently recognised histoplasmosis as a neglected tropical diseases and has included *Histoplasma* antigen tests on the WHO essential diagnostic list [30].

Histoplasmosis is a major killer of HIV-infected patients in South and Central America [29, 31]. In 2012, about 6710–15, 657 cases of symptomatic HIV-associated histoplasmosis were estimated in Latin America, with areas such as Central America, the northernmost part of South America, and Argentina having a prevalence above 30% and incidence >15 cases per 100 people living with HIV, resulting to about 671–9394 deaths related to histoplasmosis, compared with 5062 deaths related to tuberculosis reported in the region [32]. In Brazil, AIDS-associated disseminated histoplasmosis had a mortality as high as 33.1% [27]. In Guatemala, 31.2% of patients with advanced HIV had histoplasmosis [33].

Excluding the Indian sub-continent, 407 cases of histoplasmosis in South East Asia have been reported [34]. Most cases (255 (63%)) were disseminated histoplasmosis and 177 (43%) cases were HIV associated [34]. A similar study was reported from Bangladesh were 22 of the 26 cases had disseminated histoplasmosis, 4 had HIV, and 9 patients were misdiagnosed for tuberculosis [35]. In a more recent study, around 1692 cases of histoplasmosis were reported from Asian countries; India (623 cases), China (611 cases), and Thailand (234 cases) [36].

Oladele and colleagues described 470 cases of histoplasmosis in Africa between 1952 and 2017 [9]. In Nigeria, 4.4% of 750 subjects from across the country tested positive for histoplasmin skin test [13]. In the East African region, a study from Northern Tanzania retrospectively identified 0.9% cases of probable histoplasmosis among febrile inpatients, ~66.7% of whom were HIV-infected and ~77.8% were clinically misdiagnosed as tuberculosis or bacterial pneumonia [37]. In Uganda, 1.3% (2/151) of HIV-infected persons with suspected meningitis were serum *Histoplasma* IgG positive [38].

3. Syndromes of histoplasmosis

3.1 Pathogenesis

Following inhalation of *Histoplasma* microconidia, it rapidly transforms from the mycelial into the yeast form [17, 39]. Innate response involves early migration of the neutrophils toward the yeast; however, they are unable to destroy it. Alveolar macrophages then engulf the fungi but can't destroy it either, but instead the yeast multiplies inside it [17, 39]. In immunocompetent individuals, T-cell-mediated immunity is activated, and the T-cells release pro-inflammatory cytokines which activate mononuclear phagocytes, hence producing tumour necrotic factor α (TNF-α) and more cytokines [17, 39]. Well-defined granulomas are formed. *H. capsulatum* may disseminate to other organs but on activation of cellular immunity, it is quickly controlled, and individuals have a quick recovery or develop latency. Therefore, most infections go unnoticed [17, 40].

However in immunosuppressed individuals or individuals exposed to large inoculum, T-cell-mediated immunity may not contain the infection, as poorly circumscribed granulomas are usually formed, and progressive dissemination may occur [5, 41]. Patients become symptomatic and may require hospitalisation for antifungal treatment and supportive care occur [5, 41]. The most common cause of disseminated progressive disease is reactivation of latent pulmonary infection [17, 40].

3.2 Clinical manifestation

Histoplasmosis has varied presentation depending on the host immune status and the inoculum size. In immunocompetent individuals exposed to a low infectious inoculum, individuals are usually asymptomatic or experience a mild flu-like respiratory illness [41]. In most cases, these cases go unnoticed unless patients are being investigated for a suspected outbreak. Among immunocomptent travellers exposed to highly infectious (large inocula) of *Histoplasma*, acute episodes of pneumonia occurring either immediately or a few weeks later have been described [42].

Individuals whose cellular immunity is compromised for number of reasons for example HIV infection, organ transplant, immunosuppressive therapy or biological therapy, i.e., anti-TNF-α drugs usually present with a disseminated form of histoplasmosis [10, 11, 43]. Disseminated histoplasmosis presents with fever, fatigue, malaise, anorexia, weight loss, and respiratory symptoms [1, 5]. Lymphadenopathy, hepato-spenomegaly, mulluscum contagiosum like skin lesions, and oral lesions are common. Shock with multi-organ failure and coagulopathy are terminal events and are commonly misdiagnosed for bacterial sepsis [1, 5].

In acute pulmonary histoplasmosis, almost all patients are asymptomatic or experience a self-limiting infection that often goes undetected. Symptoms appear in about 10% of patients, last for less than 2 weeks and are often misdiagnosed. Such patients are usually at extremes of age, having underlying co-morbidities or immunocompromised. Common symptoms suggestive of acute pulmonary histoplasmosis include non-productive cough, dyspnoea, headache, malaise, fever, chills, and chest pain that are due to mediastinal lymph node enlargement [40]. Less common symptoms include rheumatologic complaints arthralgia, arthritis, *erythema nodosum*, *erythema multiforme*, especially in females [40]. Chest radiographs typically show diffuse pneumonitis, hilar and/or mediastinal lymphadenopathy.

Chronic pulmonary histoplasmosis includes chronic cavitary pulmonary histoplasmosis and *Histoplasma* nodule (histoplasmoma) [23]. It is a progressive disease occurring over a period of months to years. Chronic pulmonary histoplasmosis occurs in patients with structural lung diseases. Haemoptysis is common among patients with chronic pulmonary histoplasmosis, noted in up to a third of the cases. Chest radiography reveals calcified mediastinal and hilar lymph nodes of normal size along with infiltrates that evolve over time, first from focal or diffuse infiltrated to consolidations, cavitations, interstitial fibrosis, and pleural thickening, similar to patients chronic pulmonary aspergillosis and pulmonary tuberculosis [23]. Uncommon complication of pulmonary histoplasmosis includes mediastinitis, manifesting as adenitis, granulomatosis, and fibrosing [5].

Acute progressive disseminated histoplasmosis is rare except in extremes of age (less than 1 year old and more than 50 years old) and those with significant immunocompromise, for example, HIV patient with CD4 count <200 µ/l [11, 29, 32]. Acute progressive disseminated histoplasmosis may proceed after acute pulmonary histoplasmosis or re-activation of latent pulmonary lesion after a long period of latency. Patients with acute progressive disseminated histoplasmosis present with systemic (constitutional-fevers, weight loss, and weakness) and pulmonary symptoms. Focal or diffuse multi-organ is typical, with predilection for the reticuloendothelial system and the central nervous system. Physical examinations may reveal painful oropharyngeal ulceration, hepato-splenomegaly, and diffuse lymphadenopathy [5, 10, 17, 44].

4. Diagnosis

A high index of clinical suspicion is required for timely diagnosis, given the non-specific nature of presentation of histoplasmosis. A robust history, physical examination, and tailored investigation are needed simultaneously for a definitive diagnosis. Although histopathology and culture remain the gold standard for diagnosis of histoplasmosis, advancements in technology have provided *Histoplasma* antigen detection which is reliable, non-invasive, and highly sensitive [14, 41]. Misdiagnosis of acute progressive disseminated histoplasmosis has been linked to high mortality rates. Up to 42% mortality if initiation of treatment is delayed and as high as 100% if antifungal therapy is not given at all [21].

H. capsulatum can be cultured from sputum, blood, bone marrow, tissue biopsy or brochoalveolar lavage (BAL). Culture needs a period of 4–6 weeks to be appreciable as white-fluffy mould. The culture is most sensitive in patients with chronic pulmonary histoplasmosis (sputum) or progressive disseminated histoplasmosis (bone marrow) [45, 46]. Cultures have limitations such as long-turn around time, suboptimal sensitivity and require Biosafety level 3 facilities [14, 41]. Sensitivity of culture is about 70–85% [10].

Histopathology demonstrates the presence of caseating and non-caseating granulomas. Then the yeast is confirmed by special fungal stains, commonly, Gomori-methenamine silver, Giemsa or periodic acid-Schiff stains. *H. capsulatum* yeasts are about 1–4 µm in diameter, ovoid shape, predominantly intracellular (within macrophage) and giant cells with characteristic, single-celled narrow-based budding [7]. As a limitation, histopathology requires highly skilled personnel who may not be accessible across all levels of health care. Histopathology has a sensitivity of 70–80%, depending on the quality of the sample and the experience of the pathologist [10]. Because of the above limitations, we have advocated for universal access to rapid testing for histoplasmosis (antigen or PCR/molecular) [30, 47].

Histoplasma antigen detection is the most sensitive method for diagnosis. The sensitivity of the MVista® Quantitative *Histoplasma* antigen enzyme immunoassay is 95–100% in urine, over 90% in serum and bronchoalveolar lavage (BAL) antigen and 78% in cerebral spinal fluid (CSF) [10]. Sensitivity of antigen testing differs with respect to the clinical picture. A sensitivity of 91.8% in disseminated histoplasmosis, 87.5% in chronic pulmonary histoplasmosis, and 83% in acute pulmonary histoplasmosis has been reported [45, 46, 48]. Antigen testing can be used to monitor improvement on therapy, determine prognosis of patients, and ascertain possibility of relapse especially for patients with co-infections like tuberculosis [45, 46, 48]. The limitation of antigen testing is in its cross reactivity with organisms that have the same class of cell wall galactomannan such as, *Blastomyces*, *Aspergillus*, *Talaromyces*, *Coccidioides*, and *Paracoccidioides* spp. [45, 46, 48].

Antibody detection is done by different methods. The two standard assays are complement fixation and immunodiffusion [14]. Immunodiffusion detects the presence of antigens C, H and M precipitin bands. The C antigen suggests cross reactivity between fungal species; H antigen indicates active infection; and M antigen shows acute, subacute or chronic infection. Complement fixation assay generates antibody titres. The sensitivity of antibody detection by immunodiffusion or complement fixation was between 60 and 70% [10]. Immunodiffusion assay is more specific than complement fixation assay.

Polymerase Chain Reaction (PCR) assay has been widely accepted for detection of reservoirs for *H. capsulatum* in the environment [43, 49]. Bone marrow and blood specimen have high sensitivity especially in patients with disseminated disease but less in immunocompetent [50, 51]. Respiratory biopsies and samples have shown good sensitivity [14].

5. Treatment

Acute and subcute pulmonary histoplasmosis are usually self-limiting hence do not require therapy [43]. But if symptoms persist for more than a month, then oral itraconazole is given for a period of 6–12 weeks [43]. Cases of histoplasmosis-related acute respiratory distress syndrome may benefit from adjunctive corticosteroid steroid therapy.

In chronic pulmonary histoplasmosis, patients require long-term oral treatment with itraconazole for about 12–24 months or until radiological improvement on follow-up chest imaging [43]. Relapse is common following discontinuation of antifungal treatment [43].

In acute progressive disseminated histoplasmosis, induction therapy with liposomal amphotericin B for 1–2 weeks (or 2–6 weeks for central nervous system histoplasmosis) followed by a step-down therapy with oral itraconazole for 12 months [43]. Life-long oral itraconazole therapy is advised for patients with on-going immunosuppression. Liposomal amphotericin B is associated with better outcome than any other preparations of amphotericin B [52].

6. Conclusions

Human histoplasmosis is of global distribution, with patchy areas of high endemicity. The protean manifestations of histoplasmosis require a heightened index of clinical suspicion for early diagnosis and institution of appropriate treatment. Antigen-based diagnostics are the cornerstone for microbiological confirmation of histoplasmosis, given their high sensitivity and specificity, short-turn around time and non-invasiveness. Treatment is reserved for those with moderate to severe forms of pulmonary diseases, the immunocompromised, and those with disseminated diseases. Itraconazole singly or as a follow through treatment following amphotericin B are the basis of antifungal treatment.

Author details

Felix Bongomin[1*] and Lauryn Nsenga[2]

1 Department of Medical Microbiology and Immunology, Faculty of Medicine, Gulu University, Gulu, Uganda

2 Kabale University School of Medicine, Kabale, Uganda

*Address all correspondence to: drbongomin@gmail.com

IntechOpen

References

[1] Darling ST. Histoplasmosis: A fatal infectious disease resembling kala-azar found among natives of tropical America. Archives of Internal Medicine. 1908;**II**(2):107

[2] Darling ST. The morphology of the parasite (*Histoplasma capsulatum*) and the lesions of histoplasmosis, a fatal disease of tropical America. The Journal of Experimental Medicine. 1909;**11**(4):515-531

[3] Uloko A, Maiyaki M, Nagoda M, Babashani M. Histoplasmosis: An elusive re-emerging chest infection. Nigerian Journal of Clinical Practice. 2012;**15**(2):235

[4] Godwin, RA Des Prez R. Histoplasmosis. The American Review of Respiratory Disease. 1978;**117**:929-956

[5] Wheat LJ, Azar MM, Bahr NC, Spec A, Relich RF, Hage C. Histoplasmosis. Infectious Disease Clinics of North America. 2016;**30**:207-227

[6] Bahr NC, Antinori S, Wheat LJ, Sarosi GA. Histoplasmosis infections worldwide: Thinking outside of the Ohio River valley. Current Tropical Medicine Reports. 2015;**2**(2):70-80. Available from: http://link.springer.com/10.1007/s40475-015-0044-0

[7] Guarner J, Brandt ME. Histopathologic diagnosis of fungal infections in the 21st century. Clinical Microbiology Reviews. 2011;**24**:247-280

[8] Anonymous. Protean clinical manifestations of histoplasmosis. The New England Journal of Medicine. 1966;**275**(2):110. DOI: 10.1056/NEJM196607142750214

[9] Oladele RO, Ayanlowo OO, Richardson MD, Denning DW.

Histoplasmosis in Africa: An emerging or a neglected disease? PLoS Neglected Tropical Diseases. 2018;**12**(1):e0006046

[10] Myint T, Leedy N, Villacorta Cari E, Wheat LJ. HIV-associated histoplasmosis: Current perspectives. HIV/AIDS - Research and Palliative Care. 2020;**12**:113-125. Available from: https://www.dovepress.com/hiv-associated-histoplasmosis-current-perspectives-peer-reviewed-article-HIV

[11] Vergidis P, Avery RK, Wheat LJ, Dotson JL, Assi MA, Antoun SA, et al. Histoplasmosis complicating tumor necrosis factor–α blocker therapy: A retrospective analysis of 98 cases. Clinical Infectious Diseases. 2015;**61**(3):409-417. Available from: https://academic.oup.com/cid/article-lookup/doi/10.1093/cid/civ299

[12] Bezjak V. Histoplasmin tests in Ugandan sawmill workers. Tropical and Geographical Medicine. 1971;**23**(1):71-78

[13] Oladele RO, Toriello C, Ogunsola FT, Ayanlowo OO, Foden P, Fayemiwo AS, et al. Prior subclinical histoplasmosis revealed in Nigeria using histoplasmin skin testing. PLoS One. 2018;**13**(5):e0196224

[14] Buitrago MJ, Martín-Gómez MT. Timely diagnosis of histoplasmosis in non-endemic countries: A laboratory challenge. Frontiers in Microbiology. 2020;**11**(March):1-8

[15] Ashraf N, Kubat RC, Poplin V, Adenis AA, Denning DW, Wright L, et al. Re-drawing the maps for endemic mycoses. Mycopathologia. 2020:2. DOI: 10.1007/s11046-020-00431-2

[16] Richardson MD, Warnock DW. Fungal Infection: Diagnosis and Mangement. 4th ed. Oxford, UK: Blackwell Publ Ltd; 2012. p. 28

[17] Linder KA, Kauffman CA. Histoplasmosis: Epidemiology, diagnosis, and clinical manifestations. Current Fungal Infection Reports. 2019;13(3):120-128

[18] Edwards PQ, Palmer CE. Nationwide histoplasmin sensitivity and histoplasmal infection. Public Health Reports. 1963;78(3):241-260

[19] Johnson PC, Sarosi GA, Septimus EJ, Satterwhite TK. Progressive disseminated histoplasmosis in patients with the acquired immune deficiency syndrome: A report of 12 cases and a literature review. Seminars in Respiratory Infections. 1986;1:1-8

[20] Adenis A, Nacher M, Hanf M, Basurko C, Dufour J, Huber F, et al. Tuberculosis and histoplasmosis among human immunodeficiency virus-infected patients: A comparative study. The American Journal of Tropical Medicine and Hygiene. 2014;90(2):216-223

[21] Adenis A, Nacher M, Hanf M, Vantilcke V, Boukhari R, Blachet D, et al. HIV-associated histoplasmosis early mortality and incidence trends: From neglect to priority. PLoS Neglected Tropical Diseases. 2014;8(8):6-10

[22] Kauffman CA. Histoplasmosis. Clinics in Chest Medicine. 2009;30(2):217

[23] Baker J, Kosmidis C, Rozaliyani A, Wahyuningsih R, Denning DW. Chronic pulmonary Histoplasmosis—A scoping literature review. Open Forum Infectious Diseases. 2020;7(5). Available from: https://academic.oup. com/ofid/article/doi/10.1093/ofid/ ofaa119/5816327

[24] Bongomin F, Gago S, Oladele R, Denning D. Global and multi-national prevalence of fungal diseases—Estimate precision. Journal of Fungi. 2017;3(4):57.

Available from: http://www.mdpi. com/2309-608X/3/4/57

[25] Denning DW. Minimizing fungal disease deaths will allow the UNAIDS target of reducing annual AIDS deaths below 500 000 by 2020 to be realized. Philosophical Transactions of the Royal Society B. 2016;371:20150468. DOI: 10.1098/rstb.2015.0468

[26] Brown GD. Hidden killers: Human fungal infections. Science Translational Medicine. 2012;4:165rv13

[27] Almeida MA, Almeida-Silva F, Guimarães AJ, Almeida-Paes R, Zancopé-Oliveira RM. The occurrence of histoplasmosis in Brazil: A systematic review. International Journal of Infectious Diseases. 2019;62(3):261-267. Available from: http://www.ncbi.nlm. nih.gov/pubmed/31330326

[28] Nacher M, Adenis A, Adriouch L, Dufour J, Papot E, Hanf M, et al. Short report: What is AIDS in the Amazon and the Guianas? Establishing the burden of disseminated histoplasmosis. The American Journal of Tropical Medicine and Hygiene. 2011;84(2):239-240

[29] Nacher M, Leitao TS, Gómez BL, Couppié P, Adenis A, Damasceno L, et al. The fight against HIV-associated disseminated histoplasmosis in the Americas: Unfolding the different stories of four centers. Journal of Fungi. 2019;5(2). Available from: http://www. ncbi.nlm.nih.gov/pubmed/31212897

[30] Bongomin F, Kwizera R, Denning DW. Getting histoplasmosis on the map of international recommendations for patients with advanced HIV disease. Journal of Fungi. 2019;5(3):80. Available from: http://www.ncbi.nlm.nih.gov/ pubmed/31480775

[31] Disseminated histoplasmosis in Central and South America. The invisible elephant: The lethal blind spot

of international health organizations. AIDS (London, England). 2016;**30**: 167-170

[32] Adenis AA, Valdes A, Cropet C, McCotter OZ, Derado G, Couppie P, et al. Burden of HIV-associated histoplasmosis compared with tuberculosis in Latin America: A modelling study. The Lancet Infectious Diseases. 2018;**18**(10):1150-1159. Available from: http://www.ncbi.nlm. nih.gov/pubmed/30146320

[33] Samayoa B, Aguirre L, Bonilla O, Medina N, Lau-Bonilla D, Mercado D, et al. The diagnostic laboratory hub: A new health care system reveals the incidence and mortality of tuberculosis, histoplasmosis, and cryptococcosis of PWH in Guatemala. Open Forum Infectious Diseases. 2020;**7**(1). Available from: https://academic.oup.com/ofid/ article/doi/10.1093/ofid/ofz534/5678075

[34] Baker J, Setianingrum F, Wahyuningsih R, Denning DW. Mapping histoplasmosis in South East Asia – Implications for diagnosis in AIDS. Emerging Microbes & Infections. 2019;**8**(1):1139-1145. Available from: https://www.tandfonline.com/doi/full/ 10.1080/22221751.2019.1644539

[35] Rahim MA, Zaman S, Amin MR, Uddin KN, Chowdhury MAJ. Histoplasmosis: An emerging or neglected disease in Bangladesh? A systematic review. Oman Medical Journal. 2020;**35**(1):4-11

[36] Rozaliyani A, Setianingrum F. The Review of Histoplasmosis Endemicity and Current Status in Asia [Online First]. London, UK: IntechOpen; 2020. DOI: 10.5772/intechopen.92448. Available from: https://www. intechopen.com/online-first/ the-review-of-hi

[37] Lofgren SM, Kirsch EJ, Maro VP, Morrissey AB, Msuya LJ, Kinabo GD, et al. Histoplasmosis among

hospitalized febrile patients in northern Tanzania. Transactions of the Royal Society of Tropical Medicine and Hygiene. 2012;**106**(8):504-507

[38] Bahr NC, Sarosi GA, Meya DB, Bohjanen PR, Richer SM, Swartzentruber S, et al. Seroprevalence of histoplasmosis in Kampala, Uganda. Medical Mycology. 2016;**54**(3):295-300

[39] Peabody JW. Histoplasmosis. The New England Journal of Medicine. 1956;**255**(9):408-413. DOI: 10.1056/ NEJM195608302550902

[40] Kauffman CA. Histoplasmosis: A clinical and laboratory update. Clinical Microbiology Reviews. 2007;**20**(1):115

[41] Azar MM, Hage CA. Clinical perspectives in the diagnosis and management of histoplasmosis. Clinics in Chest Medicine. 2017;**38**(3):403-415. DOI: 10.1016/j.ccm.2017.04.004

[42] Staffolani S, Buonfrate D, Angheben A, Gobbi F, Giorli G, Guerriero M, et al. Acute histoplasmosis in immunocompetent travelers: A systematic review of literature. BMC Infectious Diseases. 2018;**18**(1):673. Available from: https://bmcinfectdis. biomedcentral.com/articles/10.1186/ s12879-018-3476-z

[43] Wheat LJ, Freifeld AG, Kleiman MB, Baddley JW, McKinsey DS, Loyd JE, et al. Clinical practice guidelines for the management of patients with histoplasmosis: 2007 update by the Infectious Diseases Society of America. Clinical Infectious Diseases. 2007;**45**(7):807-825

[44] Wheat J, Myint T, Guo Y, Kemmer P, Hage C, Terry C, et al. Central nervous system histoplasmosis. Medicine. 2018;**97**(13):1-8

[45] Hage CA, Ribes JA, Wengenack NL, Baddour LM, Assi M, McKinsey DS, et al. A multicenter evaluation of tests

for diagnosis of histoplasmosis. Clinical Infectious Diseases. 2011;**53**(5):448-454

[46] Hage CA, Knox KS, Davis TE, Wheat LJ. Antigen detection in bronchoalveolar lavage fluid for diagnosis of fungal pneumonia. Current Opinion in Pulmonary Medicine. 2011;**17**(3):167-171

[47] Nacher M, Blanchet D, Bongomin F, Chakrabarti A, Couppié P, Demar M, et al. Histoplasma capsulatum antigen detection tests as an essential diagnostic tool for patients with advanced HIV disease in low and middle income countries: A systematic review of diagnostic accuracy studies. PLoS Neglected Tropical Diseases. 2018;**12**:e0006802

[48] Cáceres DH, Samayoa BE, Medina NG, Tobón AM, Guzmán BJ, Mercado D, et al. Multicenter validation of commercial antigenuria reagents to diagnose progressive disseminated histoplasmosis in people living with HIV/AIDS in two Latin American countries. The Journal of Clinical Microbiology. 2018;**56**(6):JCM.01959-17. Available from: http://jcm.asm.org/lookup/doi/10.1128/JCM.01959-17

[49] Bracca A, Tosello ME, Girardini JE, Amigot SL, Gomez C, Serra E. Molecular detection of *Histoplasma capsulatum* var. capsulatum in human clinical samples. Journal of Clinical Microbiology. 2003;**41**(4):1753-1755

[50] Dieng T, Massaly A, Sow D, Vellaissamy S, Sylla K, Tine RC, et al. Amplification of blood smear DNA to confirm disseminated histoplasmosis. Infection. 2017

[51] Gago S, Esteban C, Valero C, Zaragoza Ó, De La Bellacasa JP, Buitrago MJ. A multiplex real-time PCR assay for identification of pneumocystis jirovecii, histoplasma capsulatum,and cryptococcus neoformans/cryptococcus gattii in samples from AIDS patients with opportunistic pneumonia. The Journal of Clinical Microbiology. 2014;**52**(4):1168-1176. Available from: http://jcm.asm.org/content/52/4/1168.full.pdf+html http://ovidsp.ovid.com/ovidweb.cgi?T=JS&PAGE=reference&D=emed16&NEWS=N&AN=372725898

[52] Botero Aguirre JP, Restrepo Hamid AM. Amphotericin B deoxycholate versus liposomal amphotericin B: Effects on kidney function. Cochrane Database of Systematic Reviews. 2015. Available from: http://doi.wiley.com/10.1002/14651858.CD010481.pub2

Section 2

Epidemiology

Chapter 2

The Review of Histoplasmosis Endemicity and Current Status in Asia

Anna Rozaliyani and Findra Setianingrum

Abstract

Histoplasmosis is a common disease among immunocompromised patients and a notable endemic disease among immunocompetent patients. Disseminated histoplasmosis in acquired immunodeficiency syndrome (AIDS) patients is mostly lethal. We conducted a literature review of histoplasmosis and histoplasmin skin test in Asia. There were around 1692 cases of histoplasmosis reported from Asian countries. India (623 cases), China (611 cases) and Thailand (234 cases) are detected as endemic areas of histoplasmosis although the complete mapping of this disease is still missing in some Asian countries. However, definite diagnosis is difficult since the symptoms frequently mimicking tuberculosis (TB), tissue samples are rarely obtained, and lacked of serology tests in Asian countries.

Keywords: histoplasmosis, Asia, epidemiology

1. Introduction

The first documented case of histoplasmosis in Asia was detected in a 7-year-old boy from Java, Indonesia, 26 years after Dr Samuel Darling described the first case of histoplasmosis [1, 2]. The differential diagnosis of the patient was visceral leishmaniasis, but the appendix, ileum and mesenteric lymph nodes showed histological evidences of histoplasmosis [2]. Randhawa reported 30 cases of histoplasmosis in 1970 from Asia [3]. India accounted for the highest number of 11 cases, followed by Indonesia (8 cases), Malaysia (4 cases), Thailand (2 cases), Singapore (2 cases), Vietnam (2 cases) and Japan (1 case) [3]. Together with the isolation of *Histoplasma capsulatum* from soil in Malaysia, it is implied that Malaysia is the endemic area of histoplasmosis [3]. Recent study documented 407 cases of histoplasmosis from Southeast Asian countries with Thailand as the leading country with 223 cases [4].

Human immunodeficiency virus (HIV) is a classical risk factor in histoplasmosis although there are a growing number of reports of histoplasmosis among other immunocompromised patients as well as immunocompetent patients in Asia [5–7]. The mortality of histoplasmosis among immunocompromised patients was 27.5%; this rate is significantly higher than the rate in immunocompetent patients (10%) [5]. Histoplasmosis was also often misdiagnosed as tuberculosis (TB) as many countries in Asia are high-burden TB countries [8–10]. The complete understanding of *Histoplasma* endemicity is crucial to enhance the awareness of clinicians in Asia to diagnose histoplasmosis. We reviewed the current status of histoplasmosis in Asia through analysis of published studies.

2. Methods

A literature search was conducted in PubMed and Google Scholar using the keywords "histoplasmosis" and "Asia", and also the combinations of "histoplasmosis" or *Histoplasma* or "histoplasmin" with the name of each country in Asia, in February 2020. The following countries were included as part of Asia: the Philippines, Singapore, Thailand, Vietnam, Cambodia, Brunei, Indonesia, Laos, Malaysia, Myanmar, India, Bangladesh, Pakistan, Sri Lanka, Nepal, China, Turkey, Iraq, Iran, Taiwan, Lebanon, Syria, Qatar, Saudi Arabia, Kuwait, Japan and Korea.

2.1 Epidemiology of histoplasmosis in Asia

Our review of the literature produced a total of 1692 cases of histoplasmosis reported in Asia from both areas known as endemic (Indian subcontinent, China, Southeast Asia) and non-endemic (Turkey, Iraq, Iran and Taiwan). India accounted for the highest number of cases with 623 cases, followed by China (611 cases), Thailand (234 cases), Malaysia (77 cases) and Indonesia (48 cases) (**Table 1**).

The countries included in the search to not produce any indigenous cases were Lebanon, Syria, Qatar, Saudi Arabia, Kuwait, Jordan, Japan, Korea and Brunei. Other countries in Asia were considered as non-endemic areas for *Histoplasma*, but there were possibilities of imported cases of histoplasmosis [11, 12]. Imported cases were revealed based on the travel history of patients to other Asian countries such as Malaysia, Indonesia, Thailand, Singapore and China [12]. Japan and Korea

No.	Country	No. of cases	References
1	India	623	[6, 8–10, 22–59]
2	Bangladesh	27	[6, 60]
3	Pakistan	5	[6, 61]
4	Sri Lanka	4	[6, 62]
5	Nepal	5	[6]
6	Cambodia	5	[4]
7	China	611	[7, 63–72]
8	Thailand	234	[4, 73]
9	Indonesia	48	[4]
10	Laos	1	[74]
11	Myanmar	3	[75–77]
12	Singapore	21	[4]
13	Philippines	14	[4]
14	Malaysia	77	[4, 78]
15	Vietnam	6	[4, 79]
16	Turkey	2	[16, 80]
17	Iraq	2	[18]
18	Iran	2	[19, 81]
19	Taiwan	2	[12, 20]
	Total	1692	

Table 1.
Cases of histoplasmosis in Asian countries.

revealed imported cases of histoplasmosis with 100 cases and 245 cases, respectively [13–15]. There is also small portion of indigenous cases from Iraq, Iran, Turkey and Taiwan which occurred in immunocompromised patients such as patients with long-term corticosteroid therapy, history of renal transplant or genetic immunodeficiency [16–21].

2.1.1 Indian subcontinent

The histoplasmosis cases from India are based on the study from Randhawa and Gugnani who found a total of 426 cases (1954–2018) and 207 cases from the literature search (2018–2020, excluded studies cited in Randhawa and Gugnani) [6]. The trend of reporting histoplasmosis cases was notably increased in the past 2 years, which might be caused by rising of awareness of clinicians to diagnose histoplasmosis. However, whether this increase is caused by a real increased number of patients infected by *Histoplasma* in India is unclear.

The regions along the Ganga river basins such as West Bengal and Uttar Pradesh in India were considered as endemic pockets of histoplasmosis [6, 82, 83]. Histoplasmosis cases also existed from other areas in India, which included Delhi, Rajasthan, Maharashtra and Haryana [6, 84–87]. The sole evidence of environmental source of *Histoplasma* in India was the isolation of this organism from the soil from building related to bat habitats near Calcutta, part of Ganga river basins [83].

The data of human immunodeficiency virus (HIV) status were available for 136 patients from 207 histoplasmosis patients in India between 2018 and 2020 (**Table 2**). Histoplasmosis mostly occurred in HIV-negative patients (91%, n = 124). Only 12 patients (9%) were HIV positive in this case series. The most common manifestation in the HIV-negative patients is adrenal histoplasmosis (44%, n = 54). Other study also found HIV-negative cases outnumbered HIV-positive cases with the rate of 64% proven histoplasmosis in a retrospective study from New Delhi [42].

Adrenal histoplasmosis (44%, n = 54) was the most common manifestation of histoplasmosis among 124 histoplasmosis cases with HIV negative. A recent study reported an adequate response of antifungal therapy in adrenal histoplasmosis with the rate of 86% with a median duration of follow-up of 2.5 years [50]. However, the mortality is high (20%, 8 out of 29 patients) even among patients with completed therapy.

Type of histoplasmosis	HIV positive	Reference	HIV negative	Reference
Disseminated	0	–	29	[8, 10, 22, 23, 27, 28, 33, 38, 44, 45, 47–49, 52, 53, 55, 88]
Adrenal	0	–	54	[26, 36, 43, 50, 56]
Pulmonary	1	[10]	1	[37]
Gastrointestinal	3	[24, 35]	4	[35]
Cutaneous	0	–	2	[34, 39]
Conjunctival	1	[41]	0	–
Laryngeal	0	–	1	[29]
Oral	0	–	2	[32, 33]
Mixed organs	6	[59]	31	[59]
Total	11		124	

Table 2.
HIV status from 135 patients (2017–2020) with available data.

There were no risk factors detected in 10 patients among 29 HIV-negative patients with histoplasmosis, considering this group of patients was immuno-competent [8, 10, 23, 28, 33, 44, 45, 88]. One patient had dual infections of dis-seminated histoplasmosis and TB with fever, lymphadenopathy, splenomegaly and pancytopenia [23]. The patient showed a partial response to antitubercular therapy. *Histoplasma* grew from a bone marrow culture of patient proved the diagnosis of disseminated histoplasmosis. Another unusual case was the occurrence of a progressive disseminated histoplasmosis in an immunocompetent patient with prolonged fever of unknown origin [8]. CT of the thorax was normal; later, the patient developed pharyngeal ulcer and papulonodular rash that the biopsies from these lesions turned to be positive for *Histoplasma*. The most common risk factor in HIV-negative patients was diabetes (41 patients) (**Table 3**).

A review of literature from Bangladesh revealed 27 cases of histoplasmosis with the first case reported from Dhaka in 1982. Dhaka is the most common city appeared in the list with 17 cases, followed by Chittagong, Gopalganj and Mymensingh with each of the area had one case of histoplasmosis. Four patients were diagnosed outside Bangladesh and three patients had unknown location. The cases from Bangladesh were all adult males, with 15% (four patients) who had acquired immunodeficiency syndrome (AIDS). The predominance of male popula-tion with histoplasmosis was also found in many case series [42, 50, 59]. The most common type of histoplasmosis was disseminated histoplasmosis. Seven cases of adrenal histoplasmosis in HIV-negative patients were observed in the recent case series from Bangladesh [60]. Weight loss, anorexia and fever were the common symptoms. Bilateral adrenal enlargement was seen in these patients. The diagnosis of histoplasmosis was obtained from CT-guided fine needle aspiration cytology. Four patients have diabetes as their risk factor. There is no travel history outside Bangladesh in all seven patients indicating Bangladesh as a potential endemic area of *Histoplasma*. Histoplasmosis was also reported in a small number of cases from Pakistan (five patients), Sri Lanka (four cases) and Nepal (five cases).

Several studies reported the result of histoplasmin tests in India [3, 89–91]. The range of positivity was estimated between 0 and 12.3% [3, 91]. The highest rate of positivity (12.3%) was identified from a survey in Delhi, particularly in the area near the Jumna River [89]. The zero rate of positivity was obtained from Kelur, Goa, Ramgarh and Kerala [3, 90]. The positivity of histoplasmin between 12.58 and

Conditions	No. of cases	Reference
Diabetes	41	[30, 35, 47, 48, 53, 59]
Chronic granulomatous disease	2	[52, 55]
Corticosteroid therapy	3	[9, 22, 38]
Other immunosuppressive therapies	2	[22, 38]
Idiopathic CD4 lymphocytopenia	2	[27, 35]
Kidney transplant	1	[29]
TB with severe malnutrition	1	[35]
Lymphoma	1	[35]
Chronic liver disease	1	[59]
Chronic kidney disease	1	[59]
Total	55	

Table 3.
Risk factors in HIV-negative cases from 207 histoplasmosis cases (2018–2020).

13.75% was observed among 2,729 people from Bangladesh (formerly called East Pakistan) [92]. Meanwhile, all of the 575 people (healthy participants, schoolchildren and TB and leprosy patients) showed a zero rate of histoplasmin sensitivity in Pakistan [93]. Nepal reported histoplasmin positivity in the rate of 5.7% among 1336 students and prisoners [94].

2.1.2 Southeast Asia

The total number of histoplasmosis cases from Southeast Asian countries was 410 cases with 178 (43%) cases were related to HIV-positive patients. Diabetes was noted as the risk factor in histoplasmosis case among HIV-negative patients in Southeast Asia [4]. Thailand ranked one in the number of cases of histoplasmosis in Southeast Asia, followed by Malaysia based on our literature search (**Table 1**). The dominant cases from these two countries may reflect the clinical awareness and presence of active case finding of histoplasmosis especially from HIV-positive population, which lacked in most other Southeast Asian countries [4].

HIV was found in 85% of patients in the retrospective cohort study in Thailand [95]. Risk factors for histoplasmosis were not detected in three patients (5%). Progressive disseminated histoplasmosis was the most common (86%) clinical manifestation. The organs involved include the lung, oral cavity, adrenal gland and heart valve. Most of the patients (69%) were located in Central Thailand. Weight loss, fever and anemia were commonly found in patients, followed by cough, lymphadenopathy, hepatomegaly and skin lesions. *Histoplasma* were present in microscopic examination at the rate of 89% from skin biopsy and scrape, while only 16.7% of fungal culture positive for this organism from skin tissue. The mortality rate is 12%, with all deaths coming from progressive disseminated histoplasmosis.

The evidence of environmental sources of *Histoplasma* in Thailand was obtained from the soil contaminated with bat guano and chicken dropping from Chiang Mai [96]. The detection was carried out by nested PCR on 265 soil samples. Bat guano and chicken dropping were often used as fertilizers among local gardeners. This might play a role as one of the possible contacts of this organism to humans.

A retrospective study of oral histoplasmosis in Malaysians observed older age (>54) and serious systemic illness as common risk factors [97]. All cases were proven histopathologic findings of the yeast phase of *Histoplasma capsulatum*. TB and squamous cell carcinoma were the differential diagnoses in this report. However, there is no available information regarding the immune status in this study. Five (14%) patients later developed disseminated histoplasmosis. The clinical information was not available in the remaining patients whether the patients had disseminated disease or isolated oral histoplasmosis. Other histoplasmosis cases from Malaysia were reported as a single or small case series. Disseminated histoplasmosis was diagnosed in HIV-negative patients with diabetes and high exposure of bird droppings in Sarawak, Malaysia [98]. The Malaysian Medical Association published environmental control measures to replace tall trees with shorter trees and promoted the electricity and telephone cables underground to reduce bird droppings in Sarawak [99]. The areas nearby Sarawak, Sibu and Sarikei had many histoplasmosis cases possibly due to abundant exposure of bird droppings.

Most of the histoplasmosis in Indonesia was also reported as a case report or small case series. Seven HIV-positive patients with disseminated histoplasmosis were diagnosed based on the histopathologic findings in Jakarta. The study showed there is no correlation between CD4 counts with the clinical morphology and distribution of lesions [100]. The mean CD4 count was 49.8 cells/mm3. Papules, plaques, hypertrophic scars, ulcers and scales were identified dominantly in the face. Touch biopsy was used to identify histoplasmosis in 27 patients with HIV positive in Jakarta [101]. *Histoplasma capsulatum* were detected in 10 patients (37%), suggesting this method might be suitable in the resource-limited setting to diagnose histoplasmosis.

Histoplasmin positivity in Southeast Asia varied widely across countries, ranging from 0.5% in Sarawak, Malaysia, to 86.4% in Maguee, Myanmar [4, 102–104]. Most of the studies used the induration of 5 mm or more as a sign of positive reaction. The o.5% rate was obtained from 181 schoolchildren/hospital patients, and the 86.4% rate was observed from prisoners/prison staff. Luzon Island, Philippines, reported a histoplasmin positivity rate of 26% among 143 electric company employees [104].

2.1.3 China

The number of cases from China (611 cases) was based on the recent report from Xin et al. with most of the cases reported from Yunnan province, followed by Hunan and Hubei provinces [7]. These three regions are located along the Yangtze River flows. Other provinces that are located in the Yangtze River were identified as histoplasmosis endemic regions, including Jiangsu, Sichuan and Chongqing [63]. Among the 611 cases, 34 cases from Hunan were reviewed for clinical history. It showed 13 patients were immunocompromised with most of them (8 patients) confirmed as HIV-positive cases [7]. Twenty-one patients were considered as immunocompetent. All cases were proven with tissue biopsy with the bone marrow as the most common site of biopsy. The predominant organ involved was the lungs, oral cavities and intestines.

Pan identified 300 cases of histoplasmosis in China during 1990–2011 [63]. Traveling history was present in 195 patients. It revealed that most of the patients (91%, n = 178) had no history travel outside China which indicated the endemicity of histoplasmosis in China. HIV positive comprised 22% (n = 38) of the cases among 173 patients with clear clinical information. Around 49% (n = 85) patients showed no underlying disease, with most of them (89%, n = 76) unexpectedly diagnosed with disseminated histoplasmosis.

The histoplasmin rate in normal people with no history of travel outside China revealed the highest rate is from Jiangsu (15.1%) [105]. Hunan reported a rate of 8.9%, while Xinjiang reported a rate of only 2.1%. Another study from China revealed a rate of 35% of histoplasmin positivity from Sichuan province [106].

3. Diagnostic challenges of histoplasmosis in Asia

The diagnosis of histoplasmosis in many regions in Asia is still inadequate due to the lack of awareness of this disease. Clinical symptoms are difficult to distinguish from other lung diseases, including tuberculosis and several other diseases that require different managements. The identification of *H. capsulatum* in clinical material can be determined by several techniques, including direct fungal visualization and culture, histopathology, antibody or antigen detection and molecular-based testing. These methods have different sensitivity and specificity ranges, depending upon the methodology, clinical form of the disease and host immune status.

In Asian countries with limited facilities, the diagnosis is classically carried out by direct examination of clinical specimens. The sensitivity and specificity of direct examination by using potassium hydroxide (KOH 10%) are very low. Histopathology and cytopathology with specific fungal staining is considered another important method in diagnosing histoplasmosis, but it requires invasive procedures for obtaining specimens and needs professional expertise to identify the specific fungal elements. The histopathologic examination may achieve the highest yield by evaluating bone marrow biopsies and respiratory specimens from disseminated histoplasmosis patients. A touch preparation analysis of the skin or skin biopsy shows the utility in diagnosing cutaneous mycoses or skin-related systemic mycoses, including disseminated histoplasmosis [101, 107]. The test is simple and suitable for rapid presumptive diagnosis, especially in HIV-infected patients.

4. Discussion

The histoplasmosis cases during the last 3 years in India were dominated with HIV-negative patients based on our literature search. This is in contrast with the period before 2018 that indicated HIV as the common comorbidity among histoplasmosis in India [6]. This may also reflect a decline of annual new HIV infections by 27% during 2010–2017 [108]. The endemic area of histoplasmosis in India (West Bengal and Uttar Pradesh) reported a decline of new HIV infection in 2010–2017, in the rate of 11% and 34%, respectively [108]. Meanwhile there are a limited number of studies from other regions in Asia regarding the HIV status of histoplasmosis.

Diabetes is the most common risk factor detected in HIV-negative histoplasmosis in India and Southeast Asia. India is the second country with the biggest burden of diabetes in the world [109]. There is an increase of diabetes population in India from 40.9 million people in 2007 to 77 million people in 2019 [109, 110]. The growing population of diabetes might contribute to the common findings of diabetes as a risk factor in histoplasmosis. Diabetes was commonly found as a predisposing factor in the mortality of adrenal histoplasmosis [50].

Histoplasmosis has the most varied presentations. The mild pulmonary histoplasmosis may occasionally get complicated by pericarditis or rheumatologic manifestation. After heavy exposure to *H. capsulatum* spores in the soil contaminated with bird or bat droppings, patients may present with severe acute pulmonary histoplasmosis needing hospitalization. Patients with underlying obstructive pulmonary disease may exhibit progressive chronic pulmonary histoplasmosis. Immunosuppressed patients usually present with progressive disseminated histoplasmosis, which manifests as either a chronic or acute disease. The diagnosis of *Histoplasma* which are based on tissue histopathology should be carefully evaluated as the overlap morphology of *H. capsulatum* and *Penicillium marneffei*, particularly because *P. marneffei* also endemic in certain areas in Asia [111, 112].

5. Conclusion

A rising trend of reporting histoplasmosis was observed in many areas in Asian countries. Diabetes becomes a notable risk factor among HIV-negative patients with histoplasmosis in Asia. However, the actual number of cases is still far underdiagnosed because of the lack of awareness of the clinician, minimum laboratory facilities to diagnose and the unspecific appearance of histoplasmosis often mimicking other endemic disease in Asia such as tuberculosis. Most of the studies in Southeast Asia were from a case study; a cohort study with a large number of patients is needed to reveal the clinical characteristic and evaluate the management of histoplasmosis in this region. There are an increased number of immunocompetent cases of histoplasmosis from India and China indicating that *Histoplasma* is capable to cause a disease both in immunocompromised and immunocompetent patients. There is an urgent need of proper epidemiology study of histoplasmosis to draw the actual map of histoplasmosis in Asia in order to increase the awareness of clinicians and also to facilitate early diagnosis and management of patients.

Author details

Anna Rozaliyani[1,2*†] and Findra Setianingrum[1,2†]

1 Faculty of Medicine Universitas, Department of Parasitology, Indonesia

2 Pulmonary Mycosis Centre, Jakarta, Indonesia

*Address all correspondence to: annaroza1110@gmail.com

† These two authors contributed equally.

IntechOpen

References

[1] Darling ST. A protozoon general infection producing pseudotubercles in the lungs. Journal of the American Medical Association. 1906;**XLVI**:1283-1285

[2] Müller H. Histoplasmosis in East Java. Geneeskd Tijdschr Voor Ned. 1932;**72**:889-895

[3] Randhawa H. Occurrence of histoplasmosis in Asia. Mycopathologia. 1970;**41**:75-89

[4] Baker J, Setianingrum F, Wahyuningsih R, Denning DW. Mapping histoplasmosis in South East Asia—Implications for diagnosis in AIDS. Emerging Microbes & Infections. 2019;**8**:1139-1145

[5] Gupta A, Ghosh A, Singh G, Xess I. A twenty-first-century perspective of disseminated histoplasmosis in India: Literature review and retrospective analysis of published and unpublished cases at a tertiary care hospital in North India. Mycopathologia. 2017;**182**:1077-1093

[6] Randhawa HS, Gugnan HC. Occurrence of histoplasmosis in the Indian sub-continent: An overview and update. Journal of Medical Research and Practice. 2018;**07**:71-83

[7] Lv X, Meng J, Jiang M, He R, Li M. Clinical features and endemic trend of histoplasmosis in China: A retrospective analysis and literature review. The Clinical Respiratory Journal. 2019:1-7

[8] Bauddha NK, Jadon RS, Mondal S, Vikram NK, Sood R. Progressive disseminated histoplasmosis in an immunocompetent adult: A case report. Intractable & Rare Diseases Research. 2018;**7**:126-129

[9] Dutta V, Chopra M, Kovilapu UB, Gahlot GPS. Solitary pulmonary nodule: An interesting clinical mimicry of pulmonary tuberculosis. Medical Journal, Armed Forces India. 2019;**75**:115-118

[10] Mahajan VK, Raina RK, Singh S, Rashpa RS, Sood A, Chauhan PS, et al. Case report: Histoplasmosis in Himachal Pradesh (India): An emerging endemic focus. The American Journal of Tropical Medicine and Hygiene. 2017;**97**:1749-1756

[11] Hung CC, Wong JM, Hsueh PR, Hsieh SM, Chen MY. Intestinal, obstruction and peritonitis resulting from gastrointestinal histoplasmosis in an AIDS patient. Journal of the Formosan Medical Association. 1998;**97**:577-580

[12] Lai CH, Lin HH. Cases of histoplasmosis reported in Taiwan. Journal of the Formosan Medical Association. 2006;**105**:527-528

[13] Kamei K, Sano A, Kikuchi K, Makimura K, Niimi M, Suzuki K, et al. The trend of imported mycoses in Japan. Journal of Infection and Chemotherapy. 2003;**9**:16-20

[14] Hatakeyama S, Okamoto K, Ogura K, Sugita C, Nagi M. Histoplasmosis among HIV-infected patients in Japan: A case report and literature review. Japanese Journal of Infectious Diseases. 2019;**72**:330-333

[15] Cho SH, Bin YY, Park JS, Yook KD, Kim YK. Epidemiological characterization of imported systemic mycoses occurred in Korea. Osong Public Health and Research Perspectives. 2018;**9**:362

[16] Turhan U, Aydoğan M, Özkısa T, Karslıoğlu Y, Gümüş S. A rare case in Turkey: Pulmonary histoplasmosis. Eurasian Journal of Pulmonology. 2016;**18**:116-118

[17] Yilmaz GG, Yilmaz E, Coşkun M, Karpuzoğlu G, Gelen T, Yeğin O. Cutaneous histoplasmosis in a child with hyper IgM. Pediatric Dermatology. 1995;**12**:235-238

[18] Yehia MM, Abdulla ZA. Isolation of *Histoplasma capsulatum* and *Blastomyces dermatitidis* from Iraqi patients with lower respiratory tract infections. Journal of the Islamic Medical Association of North America. 2011;**43**

[19] Pourfarziani V, Taheri S. Is pulmonary histoplasmosis a risk factor for acute renal failure in renal transplant recipients? Saudi Journal of Kidney Diseases and Transplantation. 2009;**20**:643-645

[20] Lai CH, Huang CK, Chin C, Yang YT, Lin HF, Lin HH. Indigenous case of disseminated histoplasmosis, Taiwan. Emerging Infectious Diseases. 2007;**13**:127-129

[21] Chang YT, Huang SC, Hu SY, Tsan YT, Wang LM, Wang RC. Disseminated histoplasmosis presenting as haemolytic anaemia. Postgraduate Medical Journal. 2010;**86**:443-444

[22] Bhut B, Kulkarni A, Rai V, Agrawal V, Verma A, Jain M, et al. A rare case of disseminated histoplasmosis in a patient with Crohn's disease on immunosuppressive treatment. Indian Journal of Gastroenterology. 2018;**37**:472-474

[23] Choudhury AK, Mishra AK, Gautam DK, Tilak R, Tilak V, Gambhir IS, et al. Histoplasmosis accompanying disseminated tuberculosis in an immunocompetent adolescent boy. The American Journal of Tropical Medicine and Hygiene. 2019;**102**:352-354

[24] Dawra S, Mandavdhare HS, Prasad KK, Dutta U, Sharma V. Gastrointestinal: Unusual cause of ileocecal thickening in an immunocompromised patient: A histologic surprise. Journal of Gastroenterology and Hepatology. 2018;**33**:769

[25] Gupta R, Majumdar K, Saran R, Srivastava S, Sakhuja P, Batra V. Role of endoscopic ultrasound-guided fine-needle aspiration in adrenal lesions: Analysis of 32 patients. Journal of Cytology. 2008;**5**:4-8

[26] Gupta R, Majumdar K, Srivastava S, Varakanahalli S, Saran R. Endoscopic ultrasound-guided cytodiagnosis of adrenal histoplasmosis with reversible CD4 T-lymphocytopenia and jejunal lymphangiectasia. Journal of Cytology. 2018;**5**:4-8

[27] Gupta S, Jain SK, Kumar R, Saxena R. Idiopathic CD4 lymphocytopenia presenting with progressive disseminated histoplasmosis. Medical Journal, Armed Forces India. 2018;**74**:280-283

[28] Gupta N, Vinod KS, Mittal A, Kumar APA, Kumar A, Wig N. Histoplasmosis, heart failure, hemolysis and haemophagocytic lymphohistiocytosis. The Pan African Medical Journal. 2019;**32**:1-5

[29] Jawale PM, Gulwani HV. Histoplasmosis presenting as laryngeal ulcer in a post-renal transplant male: An unusual case from India. Journal de Mycologie Medicale. 2017;**27**:573-576

[30] Kapatia G, Gupta P, Harshal M, Usha D, Rajwanshi A. Isolated lymph nodal histoplasmosis: A rare presentation. Diagnostic Cytopathology. 2019;**47**:834-836

[31] Khetarpal S, Mhapsekar T, Nagar R, Parihar A. Oral histoplasmosis masquerading as acute necrotizing ulcerative gingivitis: A rare case report. International Journal of Health Sciences (Qassim). 2019;**13**:37-40

[32] Khullar G, Saxena AK, Ramesh V, Sharma S. Asymptomatic indurated plaque on the tongue in an immunocompetent man. International Journal of Dermatology. 2019;**58**:423-424

[33] Kumar V, Bhatia A, Madaan GB, Marwah S, Nigam AS. Role of bone marrow examination in the evaluation of infections: Clinico-hematological analysis in a tertiary care centre. Turk Patoloji Dergisi. 2020;**36**:17-22

[34] Mahto S, Jamal A, Gupta P, Majumdar P, Grewal V, Agarwal N. A rare cause of nodular skin lesions with fever in an immunocompetent individual. Journal of Family Medicine and Primary Care. 2017;**6**:169-170

[35] Mandavdhare HS, Shah J, Prasad KK, Agarwala R, Suri V, Kumari S, et al. Gastrointestinal histoplasmosis: A case series from a non-endemic region in North India. Intestinal Research. 2019;**17**:149-152

[36] Muhammed H, Nampoothiri RV, Gaspar BL, Jain S. Infectious causes of Addison's disease: 1 organ-2 organisms! BMJ Case Reports. 2018:1-3

[37] Pandey M, Bajpai J, Kant S, Mishra P, Verma S. Histoplasmosis presenting as an intrathoracic mass. Lung India. 2018;**35**:41-46

[38] Pangeni R, Mittal S, Arava S, Hadda V, Ramam M, Mohan A, et al. A 44-year-old man with hemoptysis. Lung India. 2018;**35**:41-46

[39] Patra S, Nimitha P, Kaul S, Valakkada J, Verma KK, Ramam M, et al. Primary cutaneous histoplasmosis in an immunocompetent patient presenting with severe pruritus. Indian Journal of Dermatology, Venereology and Leprology. 2018;**84**:465-468

[40] Philips CA, Augustine P, Kumar L, Mahadevan P. Addison's darling crisis. Indian Journal of Pathology & Microbiology. 2017;**60**:612-613

[41] Pujari A, Rakheja V, Bajaj M, Sen S, Yadav B. Isolated conjunctival histoplasmosis in an elderly patient: A rare but important scenario. Canadian Journal of Ophthalmology. 2019;**54**:e15-e16

[42] Rajeshwari M, Xess I, Sharma MC, Jain D. Acid-fastness of histoplasma in surgical pathology practice. Journal of Pathology and Translational Medicine. 2017;**51**:482-487

[43] Ramesh V, Narreddy S, Gowrishankar S, Barigala R, Nanda S. A challenging case of pyrexia of unknown origin: Adrenal histoplasmosis mimicking tuberculosis in a patient with chronic hepatitis C. Tropical Doctor. 2018:3-5

[44] Samaddar A, Sarma A, Kumar PHA, Srivastava S, Shrimali T, Gopalakrishnan M, et al. Disseminated histoplasmosis in immunocompetent patients from an arid zone in Western India: A case series. Medical Mycology Case Reports. 2019;**25**:49-52

[45] Santosh T, Kothari K, Singhal SS, Shah VV, Patil R. Disseminated histoplasmosis in an immunocompetent patient—Utility of skin scrape cytology in diagnosis: A case report. Journal of Medical Case Reports. 2018;**12**:10-13

[46] Sethi J, Gupta KL, Mohanty T, Gupta S, Ahluwalia J, Kohli HS. Fever of unknown origin in a renal transplant recipient: Lactate dehydrogenase as an important clue to diagnosis. Experimental and Clinical Transplantation. 2019:2018-2019

[47] Sondhi P, Singh S, Khandpur S, Agarwal S. A case of disseminated histoplasmosis presenting with facial and laryngeal involvement. Indian Journal of Dermatology, Venereology and Leprology. 2018;**84**:6-15

[48] Shastri P, Gupta P. Fulminant histoplasmosis presenting as pyrexia of unknown origin in immunocompetent adult diabetic patient. Indian Journal of Critical Care Medicine. 2019;**23**:193-195

[49] Singh A, Gauri M, Gautam P, Gautam D, Haq M, Handa AC, et al. Head and neck involvement with histoplasmosis; the great masquerader. American Journal of Otolaryngology and Head and Neck Surgery. 2019;**40**:678-683

[50] Singh M, Chandy DD, Bharani T, Marak RSK, Yadav S, Dabadghao P, et al. Clinical outcomes and cortical reserve in adrenal histoplasmosis—A retrospective follow-up study of 40 patients. Clinical Endocrinology. 2019;**90**:534-541

[51] Tiwari S, Ojha S. Disseminated histoplasmosis diagnosed on bone marrow aspiration in a case of fever with thrombocytopenia. Journal of Global Infectious Diseases. 2018;**10**:112-113

[52] Abdulla M, Narayan R, Mampilly N, Kumar P. Subdural empyema in disseminated histoplasmosis. Annals of Indian Academy of Neurology. 2017;**20**:169-172

[53] Yadav A, Bansal R, Tandon A, Wadhwa N, Bhatt S. Disseminated histoplasmosis: A rare case presentation. Tropical Doctor. 2018;**48**:152-154

[54] Yadhav CSC, Elumalai K, Nishad SS, Sivannan S, Srinivasan S. Development of acrocyanosis associated with pain and increased creatinine level in histoplasmosis patient: Medication therapy. Aging Medicine. 2018;**1**:220-223

[55] Abdulla M, Mustaq S, Narayan R. Sequential surprises; non endemic mycoses revealing immunodeficiency. Indian Journal of Pathology & Microbiology. 2019;**62**:512-514

[56] Agrawal S, Goyal A, Agarwal S, Khadgawat R. Hypercalcaemia, adrenal insufficiency and bilateral adrenal histoplasmosis in a middle-aged man: A diagnostic dilemma. BML Case Reports. 2019;**12**:10-13

[57] Bansal RK, Choudhary NS, Patle SK, Agarwal A, Kaur G, Sarin H, et al. Endoscopic ultrasound-guided fine-needle aspiration of enlarged adrenals in patients with pyrexia of unknown origin: A single-center experience of 52 cases. Indian Journal of Gastroenterology. 2018;**37**:108-112

[58] Bansal N. Maltese cross birefringence in histoplasmosis. ACG Case Reports Journal. 2019;**6**:1-2

[59] Bansal N, Sethuraman N, Gopalakrishnan R, Ramasubramanian V, Kumar SD, Nambi SP, et al. Can urinary histoplasma antigen test improve the diagnosis of histoplasmosis in a tuberculosis endemic region? Mycoses. 2019;**62**:502-507

[60] Rahim MA, Zaman S, Amin MR, Nazim Uddin K, Chowdhury MJ. Adrenal histoplasmosis among immunocompetent Bangladeshi patients. Tropical Doctor. 2019;**49**: 132-133

[61] Shaikh MS, Majeed MA. Disseminated histoplasmosis in an immuno-competent young male: Role of bone marrow examination in rapid diagnosis. Diagnostic Cytopathology. 2018;**46**:273-276

[62] Sigera LSM, Gunawardane SR, Malkanthi MA, Jayasinghe RD, Sitheeque MAM, Tilakaratne WM, et al. *Histoplasma capsulatum* caused a localized tongue ulcer in a non-HIV patient—A case from nonendemic country. Ear, Nose, & Throat Journal. 2019 14556131984424

[63] Pan B, Chen M, Pan W, Liao W. Histoplasmosis: A new endemic fungal infection in China? Review and analysis of cases. Mycoses. 2013;**56**:212-221

[64] Zhu L, Wang J, Wang Z, Wang Y, Yang J, Zhu L, et al. Intestinal histoplasmosis in immunocompetent adults. World Journal of Gastroenterology. 2016;**22**:4027-4033

[65] Zhao C, Zhao S, Liu G, Xu X. Risk factors on invasive fungal infections in patients admitted to non-hematological oncology department and pediatric intensive care unit. Chinese Journal of Pediatrics. 2013;**51**:598-601

[66] Dang Y, Jiang L, Zhang J, Pan B, Zhu G, Zhu F, et al. Disseminated histoplasmosis in an immunocompetent individual diagnosed with gastrointestinal endoscopy: A case report. BMC Infectious Diseases. 2019:1-5

[67] Huang L, Wu Y, Miao X. Localized *Histoplasma capsulatum* osteomyelitis of the fibula in an immunocompetent teenage boy: A case report. BMC Infectious Diseases. 2013;**13**:1-5

[68] Liu B, Qu L, Zhu J, Yang Z, Yan S. Histoplasmosis mimicking metastatic spinal tumour. The Journal of International Medical Research. 2017;**45**:1440-1446

[69] Wang Y, Pan B, Wu J, Bi X, Liao W, Pan W, et al. Short report: Detection and phylogenetic characterization of a case of *Histoplasma capsulatum* infection in Mainland China. The American Journal of Tropical Medicine and Hygiene. 2014;**90**:1180-1183

[70] Xiong X, Fan L, Kang M, Wei J, Cheng D. Disseminated histoplasmosis: A rare clinical phenotype with difficult diagnosis. Respirology Case reports. 2017;**5**:1-5

[71] Yan Z, Xiaoli SU, Yuanyuan LI, Ruoxi HE, Chengping HU, Pinhua PAN. Clinical comparative analysis for pulmonary histoplasmosis and progressive disseminated histoplasmosis. Journal of Central South University. 2016;**41**:1345-1351

[72] Pihua G, Zhaolong C, Xinlin M, Xiaosong D, Keqiang W, Rui'e F, et al. The clinical-radiologic-pathologic features of imported pulmonary histoplasmosis. Chinese Journal of Tuberculosis and Respiratory Diseases. 2015;**38**:23-28

[73] Porntharukchareon T, Khahakaew S, Sriprasart T, Paitoonpong L, Snabboon T. Bilateral adrenal histoplasmosis. Balkan Medical Journal. 2019;**36**:359-360

[74] Jordan AS, Chavada R, Nagendra V, Mcneil HP, Kociuba K, Gibson KA. A budding surprise from the joint. The Medical Journal of Australia. 2013;**199**:700-701

[75] Hung M, Sun H, Hsueh P, Hung C, Chang S. Meningitis due to *Histoplasma capsulatum* and *Mycobacterium tuberculosis* in a returned traveler with acquired immunodeficiency syndrome. Journal of the Formosan Medical Association. 2005;**104**:860-863

[76] Murty O. Cystic tumor of papillary muscle of heart: A rare finding in sudden death. The American Journal of Forensic Medicine and Pathology. 2009;**30**:201-203

[77] Sharma R, Lipi L, Gajendra S, Mohapatra I, Goel RK, Duggal R, et al. Gastrointestinal histoplasmosis: A case series. International Journal of Surgical Pathology. 2017;**25**:592-598

[78] Marsilla MM, Khairunisa AA, Azyani Y, Petrick P. Disseminated histoplasmosis mimicking an acute appendicitis. The Malaysian Journal of Pathology. 2019;**41**:223-227

[79] Van TC, Nguyen SV, Nguyen TV, Hoang HTT, Pham PTM, Do HTT, et al. An unusual presentation of disseminated histoplasmosis in a non-HIV patient from Vietnam. Revista Iberoamericana de Micología. 2019;**36**:147-150

[80] Story H, Tennessee F, Turhan V. Tennessee (Abd)' DenTürkiye' Ye Histoplazmozun Öyküsü Histoplasmosis Story From Tennessee, USA To Turkey. Mikrobiyoloji Bülteni. 2009:339-351

[81] Aslani J, Jeyhounian M. Pulmonary histoplasmosis in Iran: A case report. Kowsar Medical Journal. 2001;**6**:21-24

[82] Kathuria S, Capoor MR, Yadav S, Singh A, Ramesh V. Disseminated histoplasmosis in an apparently immunocompetent individual from north India: A case report and review. Medical Mycology. 2013;**51**:774-778

[83] Sanyal M, Thammayya A. *Histoplasma capsulatum* in the soil of Gangetic Plain in India. The Indian Journal of Medical Research. 1975;**63**:1020-1028

[84] Malhotra S, Dhundial R, Kaur N, Kaushal M, Duggal N. Cutaneous histoplasmosis and role of direct microscopy—A case report. Clinical Microbiology Open Access. 2017;**06**:2-4

[85] Gupta N, Vyas SP, Kothari DC. Primary histoplasmosis of oral mucosa: A rare case report. International Journal of Dental and Medical Research. 2015;**1**:91-93

[86] Kriplani D, Kante K, Maniar J, Khubchandani S. Histoplasmosis in an immunocompetent host: A rare case report Dipsha. Journal of Oral and Maxillofacial Surgery, Medicine, and Pathology. 2012;**24**:106-109

[87] Sethi SK, Wadhwani N, Jha P, Duggal R, Sharma R, Bansal S, et al. Uncommon cause of fever in a pediatric kidney transplant recipient: Answers. Pediatric Nephrology. 2017;**32**:1527-1529

[88] Choudhury TA, Baruah R, Shah N, Lahkar B, Ahmed K, Sarmah BJ. Disseminated histoplasmosis presenting as oropharyngeal mass lesion. Medical Mycology Case Reports. 2019;**24**:78-81

[89] Viswanathan R, Chakravarty SC, Randhawva HS. Pilot histoplasmosis survey in Delhi area. British Medical Journal. 1960;**1**:399-400

[90] Mochi A, Edwards PQ. Geographical distribution of histoplasmosis and histoplasmin sensitivity. Bulletin of the World Health Organization. 1952;**5**:259-291

[91] Dhariwal G, Chakravarty N. Histoplasmin, coccidioidin, blastomycin, tuberculin sensitivity in relation to tropical eosinophilia and pulmonary calcifications. Indian Medical Gazette. 1954;**89**:23-28

[92] Islam N, Islam M, Muazzam M. A histoplasmosis survey in east Pakistan. Transactions of the Royal Society of Tropical Medicine and Hygiene. 1962;**56**:246-249

[93] Siddiqi SH, Stauffer JC. Prevalence of histoplasmin sensitivity in Pakistan. The American Journal of Tropical Medicine and Hygiene. 1980;**29**:109-111

[94] Uragoda CG, Wijenaike A, Han ES. Histoplasmin and coccidioidin sensitivity in Ceylon. Bulletin of the World Health Organization. 1971;**45**:689-691

[95] Wongprommek P, Chaakulkeeree M. Clinical characteristics of histoplasmosis in Siriraj hospital. Journal of the Medical Association of Thailand. 2016;**99**:257-261

[96] Norkaew T, Ohno H, Sriburee P. Detection of environmental sources of *Histoplasma capsulatum* in Chiang Mai, Thailand, by nested PCR. Mycopathologia. 2013;**176**:395-402

[97] Ng KH, Siar CH. Review of oral histoplasmosis in Malaysians. Oral Surgery, Oral Med Oral Pathol Oral Radiol Endodontology. 1996;**81**:303-307

[98] Yew Hu AS, Fong Hu AS, Hu CH. Histoplasmosis with addisonian crisis: Call for bird control. The Medical Journal of Malaysia. 2015;**70**:104-105

[99] Hu RCH. The Malaysian Medical Association's role in public health control for reduction of bird dropping hazards in Sarawak. Australian and New Zealand Journal of Public Health. 2009;**33**:194-195

[100] Sirait SP, Bramono K, Hermanto N. Correlation of CD4 counts with clinical and histopathological findings in disseminated histoplasmosis: A 10-year retrospective study. International Journal of Dermatology. 2017;**56**:926-931

[101] Wahyuningsih R, Sjam R, Suriadireja A, Djauzi S. Touch biopsy: A diagnosis method for cutaneous mycoses of AIDS patients in poor resources laboratory setting. Mycoses. 2011;**54**:89

[102] Tucker HA, Kvisseelgaard N. Histoplasmin and tuberculin sensitivity in Burma: Study of tests on 3,558 subjects. Bulletin of the World Health Organization. 1952;**7**:189-200

[103] Mardianto AT. Prevalensi histoplasmosis pada mahasiswa kedokteran Universitas Islam Sumatera Utara dan hubungan hewan peliharaan dengan tes histoplasmin. Berkala Ilmu Kedokteran. 1997;**29**:139-144

[104] Bulmer AC, Bulmer GS. Incidence of histoplasmin hypersensitivity in the Philippines. Mycopathologia. 2001;**149**:69-71

[105] Zhao B, Xia X, Yin J, Zhang X, Wu E, Shi Y, et al. Epidemiological investigation of *Histoplasma capsulatum* infection in China. Chinese Medical Journal. 2001;**114**:743-746

[106] Wen FQ, Sun YD, Watanabe K, Yoshida M, Wu JNS, Baum GL.

Prevalence of histoplasmin sensitivity in healthy adults and tuberculosis patients in Southwest China. Journal of Medical and Veterinary Mycology. 1996;**34**:171-174

[107] Held JL, Berkowitz RK, Grossman ME. Use of touch preparation for rapid diagnosis of disseminated candidiasis. Journal of the American Academy of Dermatology. 1988;**19**:1063-1066

[108] India HIV Estimations. 2017

[109] International Diabetes Federation. IDF Diabetes Atlas Ninth. 2019

[110] Sicree R, Shaw J, Zimmet P. Diabetes and impaired glucose tolerance. Diabetes Atlas. 2010:1-105

[111] Hu Y, Zhang J, Li X, Yang Y, Zhang Y, Ma J, et al. *Penicillium marneffei* infection: An emerging disease in Mainland China. Mycopathologia. 2013;**175**:57-67

[112] Chan JFW, Lau SKP, Yuen KY, Woo PCY. *Talaromyces* (Penicillium) *marneffei* infection in non-HIV-infected patients. Emerging Microbes & Infections. 2016;**5**:e19-e19

Section 3

Diagnosis

Chapter 3

Histoplasma capsulatum and *Histoplasmosis:* Current Concept for the Diagnosis

Emilie Guemas, Loïc Sobanska and Magalie Demar

Abstract

Histoplasmosis is a global deep mycosis caused by *Histoplasma capsulatum (Hc)*, a dimorphic fungus. It exists on two main varieties *Hc capsulatum* and *Hc duboisii* that could be distinguished by their epidemiology, their clinical presentation, and the morphological aspect of the fungus at direct examination of the sample. Laboratory diagnosis of *Hc* remains a real challenge as it required experience and equipment. Through a general review of literature, the different diagnosis tools for *Histoplasma* sp. are analyzed, and strengths and weaknesses are pointed according to the context-based value. Isolation of *Hc* on culture is the gold standard for diagnosis of histoplasmosis. However, it remains less sensitive (sensitivity: up to 77%) and implies long time to result, which can be inappropriate or in adapted for an emergency diagnosis. So, nonculture methods as antigen testing, serology, and molecular biology become available and allow a rapid diagnosis. However, the optimal diagnostic method depends on many parameters as the very wide range of symptomatology, the immune status. Indeed, Ag detection is the best diagnosis tool for PHD (sensitivity: 92–95%) and SCN histoplasmosis (sensitivity: 66%) and serology for the subacute/chronic form (sensitivity: 85–93%). Thus, the clinico-biological dialog is essential, and histoplasmosis management includes an integrated medical approach.

Keywords: *Histoplasma capsulatum*, diagnosis, non-culture methods, culture, performance

1. Introduction

Histoplasmosis caused by *Histoplasma capsulatum* leads to a wide spectrum of symptomatology [1–3] varying from subclinical or acute to chronic form. Histoplasmosis can be localized or it causes a disseminated, life-threatening infection involving various tissues and organs of the body, notably in immunocompromised hosts [1, 4].

This is a thermally dimorphic fungus presenting as a yeast at body temperature and as a hyaline mold in the natural environment. Human histoplasmosis is due to the two varieties of the pathogen: *H. capsulatum* var. capsulatum *(Hcc)* and *H. capsulatum* var. duboisii *(Hcd),* which could be distinguished by their epidemiology, their clinical presentation, and the morphological aspect of the fungus at direct examination of the sample [3].

Hcc, responsible for "small cell" histoplasmosis or American histoplasmosis, is well-documented in the United States mainly in the valleys of Ohio and Mississippi, South America, and Asia. Hcd responsible for "large-form" histoplasmosis or African histoplasmosis is endemic in Central and West Africa and Madagascar [3, 5–6]. We point out a third variety, *H. capsulatum* var. farcimimosum, involved in equine pathology that will not be detailed in this chapter.

Histoplasmosis can be challenging to diagnose because it is laborious and requires special characteristics for its revealing. According to the criteria recommended by the European Organization for Research and Treatment of Cancer/Invasive Fungal Infections Cooperative Group and the National Institute of Allergy and Infectious Diseases Mycoses Study Group (EORTC/MSG) and those of the Council of State and Territorial Epidemiologists (CSTE) [7, 8], an integrated approach including clinical, radiographic, and laboratory evidence is required. For laboratory diagnosis, several techniques are available as microbiology, histopathology, and immune-serological assays, depending on the clinical context and laboratory capabilities. Since 1978, the introduction of the *Histoplasma* antigen assay significantly improved the diagnosis by allowing a rapid, noninvasive, and sensitive method. Then, if culture remains the reference approach in most laboratories in endemic and non-endemic areas, non-culture methods are developing and much more improving [2, 9–11].

This review describes the current diagnostics for the laboratory identification of *H. capsulatum*, with focus on their performance and context-based value.

2. Clinical presentations and type of histoplasmosis

For Histoplasma capsulatum var. capsulatum, the inhalation of conidia from the environment (bat or bird guano) leads to Histoplasmosis syndrome or asymptomatic carriage in immunocompetent individuals. It can be self-limited especially in the lung or a progressive disseminated disease. Upon immunosuppression, the fungus can reactivate and be responsible for a localized or disseminated disease. Disseminated histoplasmosis has been classified as an AIDS-defining infection. There is a significant overlap of the pathophysiology and the clinical presentation as tuberculosis or cryptococcosis, sarcoidosis, and malignancy [1–4, 6, 12].

The histoplasmosis syndromes can be evoked according the clinical presentation, the epidemiology, and the disabled. It can be expressed as [1–2, 6]:

- A pulmonary histoplasmosis presenting as acute, subacute, chronic, or pulmonary nodules.

- A progressive disseminated histoplasmosis (PDH) that mainly concerns some particular populations (extreme age groups, immunosuppressed people including AIDS/HIV, iatrogenic origin). However, immunocompetent people defined as without obviously immunodeficiency can develop such syndrome when important inoculum.

- A cerebral nervous system (CNS) histoplasmosis.

- Other clinical findings as mediastinal histoplasmosis (adenitis, granuloma, mediastinitis).

For *Histoplasma capsulatum* var. duboisii, many features remain undiscovered as the reservoir niche, pathogenesis, and epidemiology because of the relatively low number of case reports. It expresses much more in skin and subcutaneous tissues than in lungs. Association as well with HIV is rare [5].

3. Types of specimens and context base value

All types of clinical specimens can be processed according to symptomatology [1–2, 4, 6–8]:

- Bronchoalveolar lavage (BAL), sputum, and lung biopsy should be performed for patients with pulmonary symptoms

- Bone marrow aspiration

- Punctures of lymph node, pus, or exudates

- Organ biopsies (lymph node, digestive tract, liver, skin, oral mucous)

- Peripheral blood (EDTA or fungal blood culture vacutainers)

- Cerebrospinal fluid (CSF)

Different microbiological approaches can be performed as on one hand myco-logical examination (direct, culture) and molecular assays (qPCR) and, on the other hand, histopathology. The performances depend on the specimens tested and are much more details on paragraph 5.4 (**Table 1**).

4. Direct examination for mycology

Examination of liquid smears or fine-needle aspiration and/or tissue apposi-tion on slides from all types of samples is carried out by staining with May-Grünwald-Giemsa (MGG). Using 10% KOH with or without calcofluoric acid, a chitin-binding fluorescent stain for the fungal cell wall, the yeasts can be easily visualized between slide and slip cover. For some specimens as the peripherical blood, cerebrospinal fluid, bronchoalveolar fluid, and cytocentrifugation may be required [3, 13, 14].
Diagnosis is possible according to the morphology of the yeasts.

4.1 *H. capsulatum* var. capsulatum

Yeasts are spherical, small (2–5 μm in diameter), intensely violet colored, and surrounded by a clear halo. These yeasts are narrow-based budding yeast cells, usu-ally intracellular (macrophage, histiocyte, etc.), and do not produce any filaments (**Figure 1**). The differential diagnosis includes *Leishmania* species, which is similar in size but has one kinetoplast [3, 6, 13, 14], *Candida* mainly *glabrata* and *Cryptococcus* yeast cell which is predominantly extracellular and strongly MGG stained.

4.2 *H. capsulatum* var. duboisii

Yeasts cells are oval and large (8–15 μm by 4–6 μm), with a "hourglass" or "figure eight" budding form, a thick wall and a narrow budding. They may have inside fat

		PHD	Acute pulmonary syndrom	Subacute pulmonary syndrom	Chronic pulmonary syndrom	Pulmonary nodules	Mediastinal histoplasmosis	CNS histoplasmosis	Other manifestations (pericarditis, rheumatological),
Culture	Pulmonary tissue or secretions (LBA, sputum)	x	x	x	x		(x): differential diagnosis		
	Bone marrow	x						x (if associated PHD)	
	Lymph nodes	x		(x) mediastinal					
	Exudates	x				(x) Non viable yeasts	(x) Non viable yeasts		
	Organ biopsy			(x)		x Non viable yeasts			
	Peripheral blood	x						x (if associated PHD)	
	Cerebrospinal fluid							x	
histopathology		x	x Cytopathologic examination of BAL (50%)			x Non viable yeasts	(x)		
Serology		(x)	x	x	x	X (low sensitivity)	x	X	x
Antigen		x serum, urine +/-LBA to repeat	x (83%): serum, urine +/-LBA or if associated PDH	(x) up to 40% (urine)	(x) serum, urine +/-LBA			x	

Table 1.
Preferred specimens for diagnosis according the histoplasmosis syndromes [1, 2].

(): *not preferred but can be contributive, PDH: Progressive histoplasmosis disseminated, CNS: Central nervous system, BAL: Broncho–alveolar fluid.*

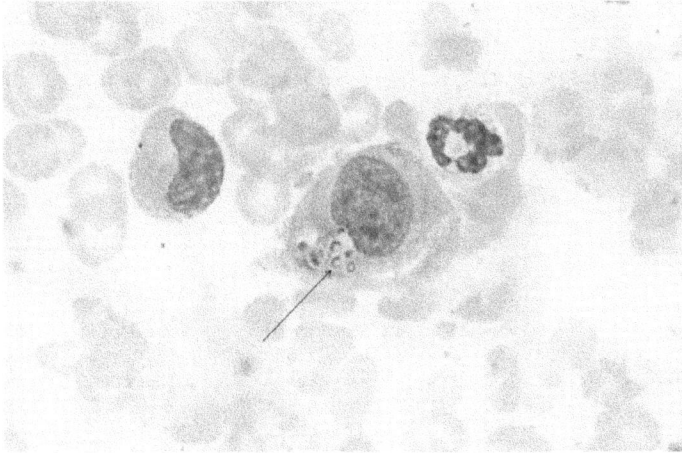

Figure 1.
Histoplasma capsulatum *var. capsulatum on bone marrow smear, intramacrophagic yeast form, microscopic appearance, magnification ×1000 (photo by Emilie GUEMAS).*

droplets. These yeasts are intra- or extracellular, sometimes arranged in short chains of 2 or 3 [3, 6, 13, 14].

Specimens as pus from abscess, draining sinuses and bone marrow lesions, colic biopsy, or BAL smears are relatively contributive to the diagnosis [4, 6, 15] in disseminated histoplasmosis.

Direct examination is inexpensive, and according to the relatively typical appearance of the levuriform elements, it allows to quickly and easily provide presumptive evidence for histoplasmosis. However, doubts may remain, and then it requires trained personnel and further investigations. Indeed confusion can concern *Hcc* versus *Cryptococcus sp., Candida glabrata*, and *Leishmania sp.* and/or if the clinical picture is not very classical [3, 6, 13, 14] or *Hcd* versus *Blastomyces dermatitidis*, which looks like another yeast cell and differs with its broad base budding.

5. Histopathology

Histopathology consists in the research for elements evocative of the yeast form of *H. capsulatum* inside tissues. Different stains can be carried out such as Gomori Methenamine Silver (GMS), Giemsa, or periodic acid-Schiff (PAS) stains that are the most relevant for the diagnosis. Hematoxylin and eosin (H&E) staining is insensitive to detect the presence of *H. capsulatum* [3, 13, 14, 16].

This concept of juggling between different stains and the description of morphologies of the microorganism (shape, size variation, cell disposition) and the tissue (cell response) permit to distinguish other pathogens as *Cryptococcus* spp., *Blastomyces dermatitis*, *Candida glabrata*, *Pneumocystis jirovecii*, *Coccidioides* spp., *Talaromyces* (formerly *Penicillium*) *marneffei*, *Leishmania* spp., *Toxoplasma gondii*, and *Trypanosoma cruzi*. These differences are represented in **Table 2**.

5.1 *H. capsulatum* var. capsulatum *(Hcc)*

It usually shows a granulomatous reaction with "giant cells," containing large rounded or oval-shaped elements (2–4 μm in diameter). *Hcc* is predominantly found phagocytosed within macrophages, histiocytes, and giant cells, often in clusters of many organisms, but sometimes they are in extracellular spaces.

	Size (μm)	Cell disposition	Characteristic	Tissue response	Specific coloration
Hcc	2 - 5	IC	Spherical with halo Narrow-based budding Grouped in clusters into macrophage	Granulamatous tissue response, necrosis	GMS, PAS
Hcd	6 - 12	IC	Oval with halo	Granulamatous tissue response	GMS, PAS
Cryptococcus	3 - 8	Facultative IC	Spherical with characteristic halo (thick capsule) Narrow-based budding	Predominantly granulomatous inflammation, necrosis, +/- fibrosis	Mucicarmin (capsulated yeast) Fontana-Masson (uncapsulated yeast)
Blastomyces dermatitis	> 15	EC	Round, Thick retractile wall Broad-based budding	Mixed suppurative and granulomatous inflammation	GMS, PAS, H&E
Candida glabrata	1 - 4	EC	Oval to round No pseudohyphal production	Suppurative tissue response	GMS, PAS, H&E
Coccidioides	2 - 5	IC/ EC	spherical Confusion when endospores are outside spherules or young spherules without endospores	Mixed suppurative and granulomatous inflammation, (Splendore-Hoëppli phenomenon likely)	GMS, H&E, +/-PAS
Pneumocystis cysts	5-8	EC	Cysts	Minimal reaction	GMS, PAS, H&E
Talaromyces marneffeï	2-5	EC	Small oval-shaped yeast Transverse septum No bud	Mixed suppurative and granulomatous inflammation	
Leishmania	2 - 5	IC	Oval to round kinetoplast		MGG

IC: *intracellular,* EC: *extra cellular,* GMS: *Gromori Methenamine Silver,* PAS: *Periodique Acid Schiff:,* GE, MGG: *May-Grunwald Giemsa.*

Table 2.
Diagnosis differential of H. capsulatum [2, 16, 13].

The yeast phase of *Hcc* is very similar to other pathogens and not distinctive in tissues from several other endemic fungi. The misidentification occurs principally with *Candida glabrata, Penicillium marneffei, Pneumocystis jiroveci, Toxoplasma gondii, Leishmania donovani*, and *Cryptococcus neoformans* [9]. However, in the appropriate clinical context, the presence of *H. capsulatum* like yeast is able to confidently make a diagnosis of histoplasmosis and is indicative of active infection. Moreover, the immunohistochemistry reaction with *H. capsulatum* antibodies can be used to confirm diagnosis of histoplasmosis.

5.2 *H. capsulatum* var. duboisii *(Hcc)*

Hcc is large (6–12 μm) and the wall is thick and highly refractive, with a pseudo-capsulated appearance. The yeast is easily distinguishable from the other endemic fungi especially *Blastomyces dermatitis* [8].

6. Culture

Isolation of *H. capsulatum* remains the gold standard for the laboratory diagnosis of histoplasmosis. However, it requires both BioSafety Level 3 (BSL3) facilities to be manipulated [17] and usually invasive methods to obtain the specimens from which culture can be performed.

6.1 Inoculation and culture of specimens

All specimen types can be used from superficial to deep ones.

Culture is performed on Sabouraud dextrose agar with antibiotics (chloramphenicol +/− gentamicin) +/− actidione that inhibits the contaminants. Other mediums can be used: brain heart infusion (BHI), yeast extract peptone agar (YEP agar) and potato dextrose agar (PDA) [3]. Mediums are incubated at 25–30°C for 6–8 weeks.

As the rate of growth is slow, the growth of the mycelial forms usually takes 2–3 weeks but may take up to 8 weeks. Colony is initially white and smooth and then becomes brown, with a granular or cottony texture. The reverse is white, yellow, or orange (**Figure 2**).

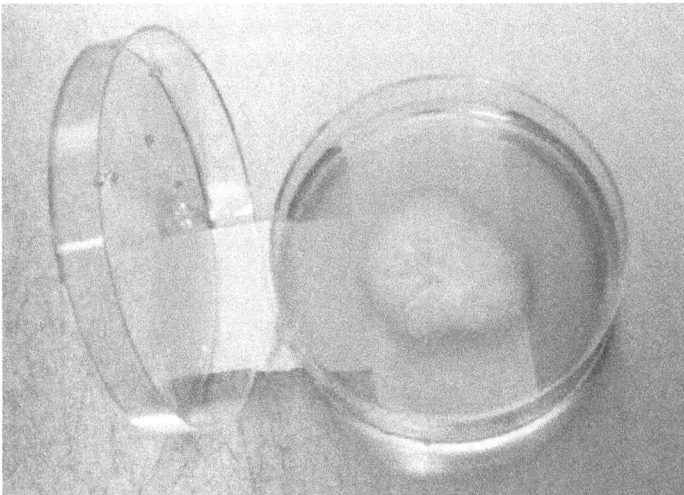

Figure 2.
Culture of H. capsulatum *on Sabouraud dextrose agar. Colony is white with a cottony texture (photo by Emilie GUEMAS).*

6.2 Identification of the fungi

Confirmation of the cultured organism as *H. capsulatum* requires complementary tests:

6.2.1 The lactophenol cotton blue test (LPCB test)

It allows determining microscopy morphology with identification characters [18]:

- **Hyphae**: hyaline septated (2–3 μm in diameter),

- **Characteristic macroconidia**: large, thick-walled, round, typically tuberculate, or knobby (7–15 μm in diameter).

- **Microconidia**: smooth-walled spherical, pyriform (2–5 μm in diameter) on short branches or directly on the sides of the hyphae

The differential diagnosis includes *Sepedonium sp.* (**Figure 3**).

6.2.2 Identification with the MALDI-TOF

The identification of the colony can be carried out by matrix-assisted laser desorption/ionization time off light (MALDI-TOF). Mass spectrometry by MALDI-TOF allows to confirm species accurately and quickly.

This identification technique is based upon the detection of highly abundant proteins in a mass range of 2–20 kDa by calculating their mass (m) to charge (z), m/z values. The spectrum thus obtained is compared with the reference spectra [19, 20].

6.2.3 The conversion from the mold to the yeast form

This can be achieved using enriched media such as BHI or blood agar plates incubated at 35–37°C in a CO_2-enriched atmosphere [3]. However, *H. capsulatum* does not convert easily depending on many parameters [13] as nutriments and temperature conditions, which can explain that this experiment is increasingly abandoned.

6.2.4 "Historic" tests

The urease test allows the distinction between Hcc and Hcd as it reveals the expression of urease strongly for Hcc and weakly for Hcd at 48 hours [3, 5].

Others tests performed from the cultured fungi such as DNA hybridization using a highly specific commercially kit (AccProbe; Gen-Probe, Inc., San Diego, CA®) or the detection of specific precipitin by the exoantigen test was used in some laboratories [10, 13]. They were gradually replaced by less time-consuming method as MALDI-TOF. They will not be more detailed in this chapter.

6.3 Blood culture

The lysis centrifugation method as Isolator® system followed by the inoculation of the collected buffy coat [11] into an appropriate media culture has been proved to be the most efficient for detecting *Histoplasma* in the blood in comparison with other methods such as conventional or automated methods such as Bactec MYCO/F

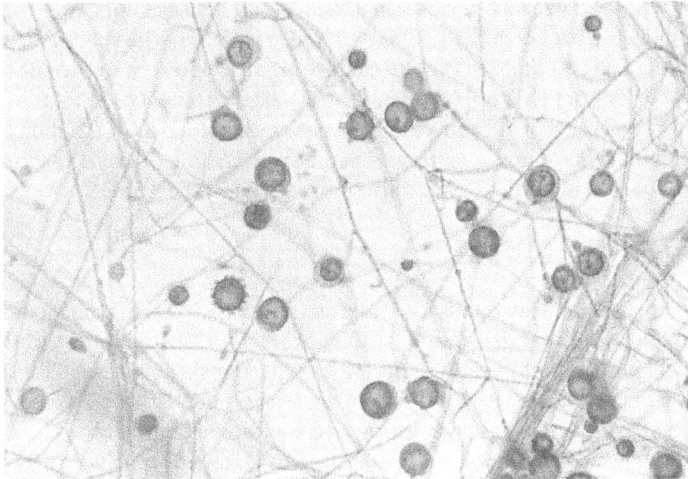

Figure 3.
Histoplasma capsulatum, *microscopic appearance with LPCB test, magnification ×400 (photo by Emilie GUEMAS).*

Lytic bottle [21]. However, many laboratories preferred those alternative systems than the manual isolator system because they permit less pre-analytic processing and continuous automated monitoring of bottles for growth when automated [9].

6.4 Performances of the culture

The sensitivity of culture depends on the clinical manifestation, the clinical specimen, the state of immunity of the host, and the burden of disease [2, 9, 14]. Sensitivity is lower for patients with acute pulmonary histoplasmosis (40%) than for patients with disseminated histoplasmosis (75%) [2, 9, 10].

The diagnosis of disseminated histoplasmosis blood culture processed by lysis methodology and bone marrow shows higher sensitivity (60–90%). Conversely, respiratory samples presented poor sensitivity (0–60%) [2, 9, 10].

The limitations of the culture are the time frame for diagnosis, the mycological expertise required, and safety. Several weeks for growth of the fungus to establish the diagnosis are not consistent with the severity of the disease in immunosuppressed patients. Moreover, *H. capsulatum* poses an infectious risk and must be manipulated in a laboratory with BSL3.

Conversely, detection of *H. capsulatum* by automated methods such as the Bactec system has not shown optimal results with sensitivity of less than 50% [2, 9–11, 13, 14] in acute and disseminated histoplasmosis that need to be rapidly diagnosed for the prompt initiation of therapy.

7. Antibody detection

Several protocols do exist based on *Histoplasma*-specific antibody detection with three routinely used assays: immunodiffusion test (ID), fixation complement test (FC), and indirect immunological assays (EIA) [9–11, 13, 14, 22–26]. Serology aims to confirm a previously contact with the pathogen, and it usually does not mean that the patient is making an acute infection. For histoplasmosis, in certain circumstances, serology can detect the acute phase of histoplasmosis. It is reported that the antibodies detection period is between 4 and 8 weeks but can be negative in immunodeficient patients [10, 14]. The serologic targets are the specific *Histoplasma* proteins M (a catalase) and H (a β-glucosidase) that are present in the entire yeast or an antigenic extract (histoplasmin or HMIN) used as deglycosylate or not, from mycelial culture. Another protein can be targeted, the protein C (a carbohydrate, galactomannan), that is less specific and can be responsible of cross-reactions with other fungi [9]. Their characteristics are summarized in the **Table 3**.

7.1 Immunodiffusion (ID)

Immunodiffusion assay qualitatively detects the precipitating antibodies to antigens M and H on agar gel. The H band appears after the M band, and the presence of both bands is highly significant for histoplasmosis diagnosis. Thus, M band is detectable in most patients with acute infection and persists for long periods of time up to 3 years after disease resolution and is often present in chronic forms [9, 10, 14]. It does not distinct between active from latent or resolved infection. H band is less frequent, confirms acute infection only in 7% according [13], remains present 1–2 years after disease resolution, and indicates a more severe form of the disease. This method is simple, reliable, and inexpensive.

7.2 Complement fixation (FC)

Complement fixation method quantitatively measures the presence of complex antigen antibodies in a patient's serum against the entire yeast form or mycelial antigen (HMIN) from 3 to 6 weeks following infection [13]. Interlaboratory results vary as it is entirely strain-dependent for the antigen preparation. It is quite more sensitive bus less specific than the ID. Indeed, it presents numerous cross-reactions with other fungi and interference with rheumatoid factor and cold agglutinins [13]. A threshold defined as up to 1:32 or titer a 4-fold rise indicates an active infection.

7.3 Enzyme-linked immunosorbent assay (ELISA)

This method does not allow differentiation between an active infection and an old infection. Indeed, antibodies require 4–8 weeks to become detectable in peripheral blood. Serology is unreliable in patients with a reduced ability to produce antibodies, and then it is often negative in immunocompromised patients [13, 14]. Antibody testing is most useful for subacute and chronic forms of histoplasmosis [2].

7.4 Western blot

Western blot immunoassay uses Ag proteins of different kDa that will complex with the specific *Histoplasma* antibodies on a nitrocellulose band. It showed good results but does not exist as a commercial kit, so it can be fastidious to set up. The sensibility is improved by the treatment of the Ag (Histoplasmin) [22].

7.5 Other tests

Interferon gamma release assay (IGRA): this test is based on the quantification of lymphocyts-released interferon (IFN) -γ after restimulation in vitro of the cell-mediated immunity with the same specific antigens. Recently, Rubio-Carrasquilla et al. [23] considered it as a promising screening method to detect individuals with latent Hc infection, even decades after the primary infection.

	Complement fixation (FC)	Immunodiffusion (ID)	ELISA	Western Blott
Mechanisms	A supplemented specific Ag induces Ag-Ab complexes	Precipitins Ac-Ag (H/M) on gel agar	Indirect sandwich ELISA	Visualisation of band profiles on nitrocellulose membranes
Type of Ag	Entire yeast or HMIN	HMIN Prot M, Prot H	Yeast cell extract, ribosome, HMIN (glycosylayte/ deglycosylate)	Histoplasma antigens of 115, 91,88, 83, 70 and 38 kDa from HMIN (glycosylayte/deglycosylate)
delay	3 -6 weeks	4-6 weeks IgG anti-M → IgG M+H	2 -4 weeks	2-4 weeks
Duration of positive antibodies after resolution	Months to years Months to years Persistent in recurrences	Prot M: up to 3 years Prot H: 1-2 years	Months to years	Months to years
Sensitivity	72-95%	70-95%	75-100%	45-100%
Specificity	70-80%	100%	91-100%	94-100%
Histoplasmosis meningitidis	When positive (culture usually negative (63%)	When positive (culture usually negative (44%)	Specificity: 93% Sensibility: 82% (26)	No data
Acute infection	++	Band M (80%) Band H (7-20%)	66-100% (9-10, 13)	45-94% (13, 22)
Chronic infection	+	Band M	90% (9-10, 13)	94-100% (13, 22)
Special remarks	Interference with Rheumatoid factor and cold agglutinins	Positive after skin test Histoplasmine (M ++/H+)	Ribosome antigen and ptHMIN induces better response than glycosylate HMIN antigene. Best results with ELISA using ferrous metal	Better results when using ptHMIN Can detect early in the infection
Kits/tests	House-made tests	House-made tests	House-made tests Commercialized tests with IgG, IgM, IgA	House-made tests

Histoplasmine : HMIN, deglycosylated HMIN: tptHMIN.

Table 3.
Summary of serological assays [2, 9, 10, 13, 14, 22, 26].

Latex agglutination tests were developed as a commercial kit, but false positives results were found in patients with tuberculosis. It was compared as more sensitive than CF [13].

A hemagglutination test was available but failed to differentiate *B. dermatitidis* [13].

A recent meta-analysis [9] interested in the global sensitivity of antibody detection for disseminated histoplasmosis and showed a low sensitivity of 58% in contrast with high specificity (100%). But there is a real distinction between the different assays. WB and ELISA methods have the highest analytical performance, with sensitivity of up to 90% when used in ptHMIN. This can explain that it is relevant to associate different methods in order to improve the diagnosis.

Cross-reactivity with granulomatous disease, tuberculosis, and sarcoidosis can occur with immunodiffusion and complement fixation tests. Moreover, serologic cross-reaction can occur with other common fungal pathogens like *Blastomyces dermatitidis*, *Coccidioides immitis*, *Aspergillus fumigatus*, and *Paracoccidioides brasiliensis* [24, 25].

The presence of antibodies in the CSF allows making the diagnosis of Histoplasma meningitis [2, 26].

8. Antigen detection

8.1 Target antigens

8.1.1 Specific-Histoplasma *antigen detection*

Circulating specific-*Histoplasma* polysaccharide antigen (HPA) detection is a useful option for diagnosis [9, 13–14, 27–28]. *Histoplasma* galactomannan is the target of the antigenic detection. Since its introduction in 1986 [13–14], as a solid-phase radioimmunoassay, it was developed into a sandwich enzyme immunoassay (EIA) [2, 13, 27–29] with different improved generations and recently into a lateral flow assay (LFA) [30]. Their performance is related to the choice of the antibodies used monoclonal versus polyclonal, and the conjugate (Biotine or horseradish peroxidase) [13].

8.1.2 Galactomannan antigen detection

This polysaccharide mostly found in the cell wall of *Aspergillus* sp. is commonly used for invasive aspergillosis diagnosis in high-risk immunosuppressed patients suffering of solid organ transplantation or hematological malignancies. Cross-reactivity with the histoplasma antigen detection is reported suggesting that this test could be a potentially helpful diagnostic test for histoplasmosis in HIV-infected patient because of the low incidence of invasive aspergillosis in this population. The sensibility of this test for diagnosis of disseminated histoplasmosis in AIDS patients is 77% and specificity is 100% [31].

8.2 Technical methods

8.2.1 Enzyme immunoassay (EIA)

This noninvasive method can be performed in urine, serum, and other body fluids as LBA [2, 9, 10, 13–14] and is the simplest diagnostic method, easily implemented in low- and middle-income countries.

It allows a rapid diagnosis especially for immunosuppressed patients with severe acute or disseminated histoplasmosis. It is less sensitive than serology for the diagnosis of subacute and chronic pulmonary histoplasmosis [2, 9].

Antigen detection in urine is more sensitive than in serum for the diagnosis of disseminated histoplasmosis (95% versus 86% for HIV-infected patient) [9, 10–11]. However, antigen detection in urine is less useful for pulmonary forms or chronic histoplasmosis.

This method has also been applied to other body fluids, including BAL for patient with pulmonary symptomatology and CSF for *Histoplasma* meningitis. Antigen was detected in the CSF of 66% of immunosuppressed-infected patient patients who had *Histoplasma* meningitis [26].

If useful for the diagnosis, it can also monitor the antigen clearance, particularly in serum and thus appears as an useful marker for treatment response [32].

Moreover, it has proven its applicability to infected animals that may act as potential reservoirs for humans [28, 29].

Cross-reactivity of antigen testing occurs in patients who have other fungal infections, including infections by *Blastomyces dermatitidis, Paracoccidioides brasiliensis,* and *Penicillium marneffei* [33]. The most problematic issue is differentiating histoplasmosis and blastomycosis because the geographic areas overlap.

8.2.2 Lateral flow assay (LFA)

Recently, a lateral flow assay (LFA) has been developed and evaluated for rapid diagnosis of histoplasmosis. This point of care antigen detection in serum allows rapid results with high analytical performance. It is based on the using of rabbit polyclonal antibody that recognizes galactomannan antigen of *H. capsulatum.* Indeed, sensitivity is under 95% and specificity is 90%. Cross-reactivity occurs principally with paracoccidioidomycosis [30].

9. Molecular tests

9.1 Polymerase chain reaction (PCR)

Molecular methods can improve and accelerate the histoplasmosis diagnosis with a high analytical sensibility and specificity [9, 10, 34–36]. This combined with turnaround times shorter than those of other diagnostics. It is much more safety and reduces the risk of laboratory acquired histoplasmosis when handle its positive culture. Several applications can be linked to the use of PCR based techniques as (i) human diagnosis from different samples, with an increasingly use for the imported cases diagnosis in non-endemic areas [9–11, 13], (ii) environmental exploration for revealing the histoplasmosis reservoir [35], (iii) and prevention policies and strategies for exposure risk [2].

There are no currently official approved molecular assays for H. capsulatum that are directly applicable to clinical specimens and no commercially kits are available [9, 10, 34]. However, there are numerous reports of the laboratory-developed PCR assays (in house PCR) using the different type of PCR (conventional, nested and quantitative) and a variety of molecular targets. The most relevant are the Internal Transcribed Spacer (ITS) multicopy region of the ribosomal DNA, genes encoding the M antigen or the 100-kDa-like protein [9, 34]. Most studies in the literature evaluated the performance of nested PCR in the diagnosis of PDH, this assay is associated with the increased risk of amplicon contamination, because of the manipulation of amplified products.

A multiplex approach can also be performed. For example, in a reference laboratory in Spain they developed a multiplex qPCR for *H. capsulatum, Pneumocystis jirovecii* and *Cryptococcus neoformans* [11].

As a full tool to Histoplasmosis diagnosis, molecular assays can be performed on different types of specimens including respiratory secretions, biopsies, bone marrow, blood, or sera.

For diagnosis of disseminated histoplasmosis (PDH), sensitivity and specificity are 95% and 99%, respectively [2, 9]. Sample of blood and bone marrow have an excellent sensitivity (100%) in immunocompromised patients with disseminated histoplasmosis, whereas it is weaker in immunocompetent patients [2, 11].

Moreover, sensitivity increases by testing more than one sample per patient in cases with extra-pulmonary histoplasmosis. So, in case of high suspicion, clinicians should repeat and diversify samples [2, 9, 11, 34].

Recent findings in molecular biology permit to evaluate genetic diversity using multilocus sequence typing (MLST) OR RAPD-PCR [36]. This could be Interesting to associate genotypes and clinical presentation.

9.2 Loop-mediated isothermal amplification (LAMP)

9.2.1 Principe

Loop-mediated isothermal amplification (LAMP) is a highly efficient, sensitive, specific and cost-effective isothermal amplification method that uses at least four primers, recognizing six different regions in the target sequence (**Figure 4**) and results in a self-primed DNA [37].

In LAMP, the target sequence is amplified at a constant temperature of 60–65°C using either two or three sets of primers and a polymerase with high strand displacement activity in addition to a replication activity. The amount of DNA produced in LAMP is considerably higher than PCR-based amplification.

To increase the reaction sensitivity, the ITS region was used as target, since it is a multicopy sequence and also because it is considered an important barcoding sequence for fungal identification, being conserved among *H. capsulatum* strains and divergent from other fungi, ensuring high specificity.

Forward inner primer (FIP) and backward inner primer (BIP) have inverted sequences attached at the 5′ end, named F1c and B1c, which are complementary to an internal sequence from the amplified strand, forming a loop at each extremity of a single strand DNA.

The outer primers (F3 and B3) anneal upstream to the FIP and BIP, acting as a binding site for DNA polymerase, which, in the LAMP reaction, also contains the strand displacement activity.

LAMP results can be observed using several strategies with minimal ambiguity with real-time turbidimetry (magnesium pyrophosphate formation), fluorescent compounds (Sybr Green, Eva Green, SYTO, calcein), magnesium colorimetric titration, fluorescent-labeled probes, quencher-labeled primers, dye-labeled primers, and PH-sensitive dyes.

9.2.2 Indications

LAMP can be used on samples of whole blood or bone marrow for patients suspected of progressive disseminated histoplasmosis (PDH).

A new assay, the so-called ITS LAMP, showed no cross-reactivity when assayed with DNA from other pathogenic or environmental fungi. The assay is able to detect isolates from all geographical clades of *H. capsulatum*, including Hcd. In comparison with Hcp100 nPCR, it reached sensitivity of 83% and specificity of 92% [35].

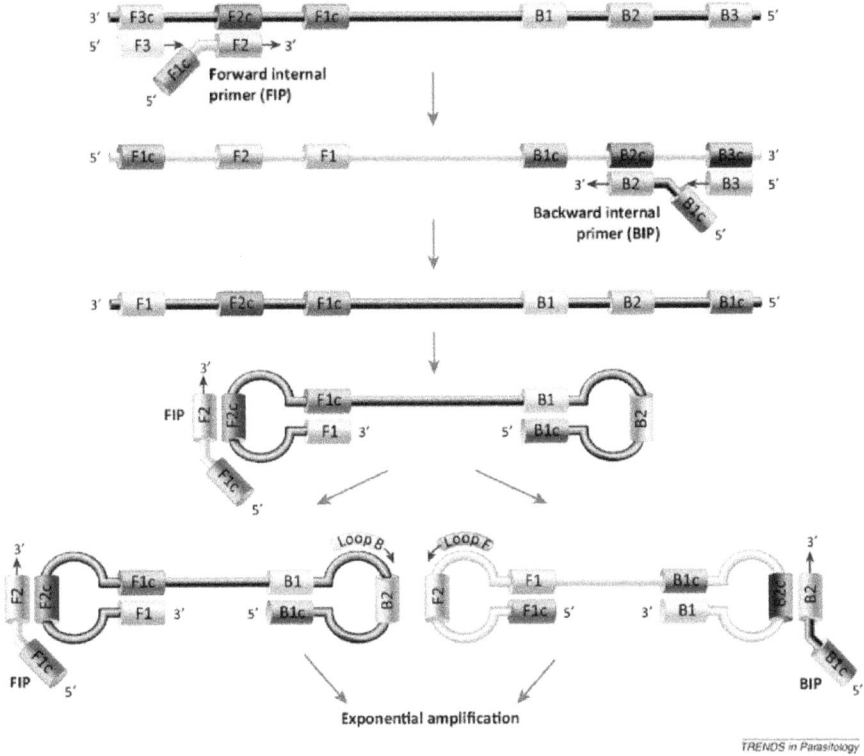

Figure 4.
Principe of LAMP [38].

This method remains cost-effective with or without the extraction DNA step and did not require a thermocycler or an electrophoresis apparatus. It saves time with test performed in less than 200 minutes [35]. However, this little-known and recent method is currently underused and much more reserved for resource-limited laboratories. It should evolve in the next years to come and need further evaluation to be routinely used.

10. Summary of the different categories of tests and their sensitivity (%)

The performance for each test according the clinical context is summarized in **Table 4**. It considers global sensitivity without any distinction between the different protocols (antigen preparation, methods, …).

It highlights that Ag detection is the best diagnosis tool for PHD and SCN histoplasmosis, serology for the subacute/chronic form, and the culture although this is the reference method remains less sensitive.

11. Conclusion

Histoplasmosis remains a severe and neglected disease for which early diagnosis of invasive fungal infections is critical to allow a prompt patient care. Indeed the mortality rate among HIV/AIDS patients diagnosed with histoplasmosis is high: 42% mortality for disseminated histoplasmosis if treatment is delayed and 100% if antifungal therapy is not prescribed.

	PHD (2)	PHD (9)	Acute pulmonary syndrom	Subacute pulmonary syndrom	Chronic pulmonary syndrom	Mediastinal histoplasmosis	CNS histoplasmosis	
Ag detection	92	95	83	30	88	5	66	
							81	31
Serology	75	58	64	95	83	83	59	
							63	54
Pathology	76	NE	20	42	75	75		
culture	74	77	42	54	67	67	38	
							40	33
Molecular Biology		95						

PDH: Progressive histoplasmosis disseminated, CNS: Central nervous system, NE: Non evaluated.

Table 4.
The different performances (sensibilité %)of the methods are summarized in this table adapted to azar et al. (2), Caceres et.al (9) and Wheat et.al (26).

The gold standard for histoplasma diagnosis remains culture. It's a time-consuming process and has limitations in sensitivity. Moreover, it requires invasive procedure and mycological expertise.

Nonculture methods have been developed to improve and accelerate diagnosis of histoplasmosis, such as histoplasma antigen detection, antibody detection, and molecular biology. It should have conjunction between the different tools of diagnosis to be reliable in the histoplasmosis management regarding the wide range of clinical features.

Author details

Emilie Guemas[1], Loïc Sobanska[1] and Magalie Demar[1,2*]

1 Academic Laboratory of Parasitology and Mycology, Cayenne Hospital, French Guiana

2 Amazonian Ecosystem and Tropical Diseases (EA 3593, EPat), University of French Guiana, Cayenne, French Guiana

*Address all correspondence to: magalie.demar@ch-cayenne.fr

IntechOpen

References

[1] Wheat LJ, Freifeld AG, Kleiman MB, et al. Clinical practice guidelines for the management of patients with histoplasmosis: 2007 update by the Infectious Diseases Society of America. Clinical Infectious Diseases. 2007;45(7):807-825. DOI: 10.1086/521259

[2] Azar MM, Loyd JL, Relich RF, Wheat LJ, Hage CA. Current concepts in the epidemiology, diagnosis, and Management of Histoplasmosis Syndromes. Seminars in Respiratory and Critical Care Medicine. 2020;41(1): 13-30. DOI: 10.1055/s-0039-1698429

[3] Société Française de Microbiologie. Chromoblastomycose et Histoplasmose. In: Rémic. Paris: Société française de microbiologie; 2018. pp. 911-926

[4] Couppié P, Herceg K, Bourne-Watrin M, et al. The broad clinical Spectrum of disseminated Histoplasmosis in HIV-infected patients: A 30 Years' experience in French Guiana. Journal of Fungi. 2019;5(4):115. DOI: 10.3390/jof5040115

[5] Valero C, Gago S, Monteiro MC, Alastruey-Izquierdo A, Buitrago MJ. African histoplasmosis: New clinical and microbiological insights. Medical Mycology. 2018;56(1):51-59. DOI: 10.1093/mmy/myx020

[6] Oladele RO, Ayanlowo OO, Richardson MD, Denning DW. Histoplasmosis in Africa: An emerging or a neglected disease? PLoS Neglected Tropical Diseases. 2018;12(1):e0006046. DOI: 10.1371/journal.pntd.0006046

[7] De Pauw B, Walsh TJ, Donnelly JP, Stevens DA, Edwards JE, Calandra T, et al. Revised definitions of invasive fungal disease from the European Organization for Research and Treatment of cancer/invasive fungal infections cooperative group and the National Institute of Allergy and Infectious Diseases mycoses study group (EORTC/MSG) consensus group. Clinical Infectious Diseases. 2008;46(12):1813-1821

[8] CDC. Histoplasmosis 2017 case definition [Internet]. Available from: https://wwwn.cdc.gov/nndss/conditions/histoplasmosis/case-definition/2017

[9] Caceres DH, Knuth M, Derado G, Lindsley MD. Diagnosis of progressived disseminated histoplasmosis in advanced HIV: A meta-analysis of assay analytical performance. Journal of Fungi. 2019;5(3):76

[10] Scheel CM, Gómez BL. Diagnostic methods for Histoplasmosis: Focus on endemic countries with variable infrastructure levels. Current Tropical Medicine Reports. 2014;1(2):129-137. DOI: 10.1007/s40475-014-0020-0

[11] Buitrago MJ, Martín-Gómez MT. Timely diagnosis of Histoplasmosis in non-endemic countries: A laboratory challenge. Frontiers in Microbiology. 2020;11:467. DOI: 10.3389/fmicb.2020.00467

[12] Caceres DH, Valdes A. Histoplasmosis and tuberculosis co-occurrence in people with advanced HIV. Journal of Fungi. 2019;5(3):73. DOI: 10.3390/jof5030073

[13] Guimarães AJ, Nosanchuk JD, Zancopé-Oliveira RM. Diagnosis of histoplasmosis. Brazilian Journal of Microbiology. 2006;37(1):1-13. DOI: 10.1590/S1517-83822006000100001

[14] Azar MM, Hage CA. Laboratory diagnostics for histoplasmosis. Journal of Clinical Microbiology. 2017;55(6):1612-1620

[15] Adenis AA, Aznar C, Couppié P. Histoplasmosis in HIV-infected patients:

A review of new developments and remaining gaps. Current Tropical Medicine Reports. 2014;**1**(2):119-128

[16] Guarner J, Brandt ME. Histopathologic diagnosis of fungal infections in the 21st century. Clinical Microbiology Reviews. 2011;**24**(2): 247-280. DOI: 10.1128/CMR.00053-10

[17] Kauffman CA. Histoplasmosis: A clinical and laboratory update. Clinical Microbiology Reviews. 2007;**20**(1):115-132

[18] Guimarães AJ, de Cerqueira MD, Nosanchuk JD. Surface architecture of *Histoplasma capsulatum*. Frontiers in Microbiology. 18 November 2011;**2**:225. DOI: 10.3389/fmicb.2011.00225

[19] Valero C, Buitrago MJ, Gago S, Quiles-Melero I, García-Rodríguez J. A matrix-assisted laser desorption/ ionization time of flight mass spectrometry reference database for the identification of *Histoplasma capsulatum*. Medical Mycology. 2018;**56**(3):307-314. DOI: 10.1093/mmy/myx047

[20] Rychert J, Slechta ES, Barker AP, et al. Multicenter evaluation of the Vitek MS v3.0 system for the identification of filamentous fungi. Journal of Clinical Microbiology. 24 January 2018;**56**(2):e01353-17. DOI: 10.1128/ JCM.01353-17

[21] Vetter E, Torgerson C, Feuker A, et al. Comparison of the BACTEC MYCO/F lytic bottle to the isolator tube, BACTEC plus aerobic F/bottle, and BACTEC anaerobic lytic/10 bottle and comparison of the BACTEC plus aerobic F/bottle to the isolator tube for recovery of bacteria, mycobacteria, and fungi from blood. Journal of Clinical Microbiology. 2001;**39**(12):4380-4386. DOI: 10.1128/JCM.39.12.4380-4386.2001

[22] de Almeida MA, Pizzini CV, Damasceno LS, de Muniz M, Almeida-Paes R, RHS P, et al. Validation of western blot for *Histoplasma capsulatum* antibody detection assay. BMC Infectious Diseases. 2016;**16**(1):87

[23] Rubio-Carrasquilla M, Santa CD, Rendón JP, et al. An interferon gamma release assay specific for Histoplasma capsulatum to detect asymptomatic infected individuals: A proof of concept study. Medical Mycology. 2019;**57**(6):724-732. DOI: 10.1093/mmy/ myy131

[24] Wheat J, French ML, Kamel S, Tewari RP. Evaluation of cross-reactions in Histoplasma capsulatum serologic tests. Journal of Clinical Microbiology. 1986;**23**(3):493-499

[25] Negroni R, De Flores CI, Robles AM. Study of serologic cross reactions between the antigens of Paracoccidioides brasiliensis and Histoplasma capsulatum. Revista de la Asociación Argentina de Microbiología. 1976;**8**(2):68-73

[26] Wheat J, Myint T, Guo Y, et al. Central nervous system histoplasmosis: Multicenter retrospective study on clinical features, diagnostic approach and outcome of treatment. Medicine (Baltimore). 2018;**97**(13):e0245. DOI: 10.1097/MD.0000000000010245

[27] Zhang X, Gibson B, Daly TM. Evaluation of commercially available reagents for diagnosis of histoplasmosis infection in immunocompromised patients. Journal of Clinical Microbiology. 2013;**51**(12):4095-4101

[28] Cunningham L, Cook A, Hanzlicek A, Harkin K, Wheat J, Goad C, et al. Sensitivity and specificity of Histoplasma antigen detection by enzyme immunoassay. Journal of the American Animal Hospital Association. 2015;**51**(5):306-310

[29] Rothenburg L, Hanzlicek AS, Payton ME. A monoclonal antibody-based urine Histoplasma antigen

enzyme immunoassay (IMMY®) for the diagnosis of histoplasmosis in cats. Journal of Veterinary Internal Medicine. 2019;**33**(2):603-610

[30] Cáceres DH, Gómez BL, Tobón AM, Chiller TM, Lindsley MD. Evaluation of a Histoplasma antigen lateral flow assay for the rapid diagnosis of progressive disseminated histoplasmosis in Colombian patients with AIDS. Mycoses. 2020;**63**(2):139-144

[31] Iriart X, Blanchet D, Menard S, Lavergne R-A, Chauvin P, Adenis A, et al. A complementary tool for management of disseminated Histoplasma capsulatum var. capsulatum infections in AIDS patients. International Journal of Medical Microbiology. 2014;**304**(8):1062-1065

[32] Myint T, Anderson AM, Sanchez A, Farabi A, Hage C, Baddley JW, et al. Histoplasmosis in patients with human immunodeficiency virus/ acquired immunodeficiency syndrome (HIV/AIDS): Multicenter study of outcomes and factors associated with relapse. Medicine (Baltimore). 2014;**93**(1):11-18

[33] Wheat LJ. Improvements in diagnosis of histoplasmosis. Expert Opinion on Biological Therapy. 2006;**6**(11):1207-1221

[34] Vasconcellos ICDS, Dalla Lana DF, Pasqualotto AC. The role of molecular tests in the diagnosis of disseminated Histoplasmosis. Journal of Fungi. 2019;**6**(1):1. DOI: 10.3390/jof6010001

[35] Gómez LF, Arango M, McEwen JG, et al. Molecular epidemiology of Colombian Histoplasma capsulatum isolates obtained from human and chicken manure samples. Heliyon. 2019;**5**(7):e02084. DOI: 10.1016/j.heliyon.2019.e02084

[36] Sahaza JH, Duarte-Escalante E, Canteros C, Rodríguez-Arellanes G, Reyes-Montes MR, Taylor ML. Analyses of the genetic diversity and population structures of Histoplasma capsulatum clinical isolates from Mexico, Guatemala, Colombia and Argentina, using a randomly amplified polymorphic DNA-PCR assay. Epidemiology and Infection. 2019;**147**:e204. DOI: 10.1017/S0950268819000931

[37] da Zatti MS, Arantes TD, Fernandes JAL, Bay MB, Milan EP, Naliato GFS, et al. Loop-mediated isothermal amplification and nested PCR of the internal transcribed spacer (ITS) for Histoplasma capsulatum detection. PLoS Neglected Tropical Diseases. 2019;**13**(8):e0007692

[38] Alhassan A, Li Z, Poole CB, Carlow CKS. Expanding the MDx toolbox for filarial diagnosis and surveillance. Trends in Parasitology. 2015;**31**(8):391-400

Chapter 4

Laboratory Diagnosis of Histoplasmosis: An Update

María J. Buitrago and Clara Valero

Abstract

Early diagnosis of histoplasmosis is essential to establish a suitable antifungal therapy and reduce morbidity and mortality rates. However, laboratory diagnosis remains challenging due to the low availability of proper methods and the lack of clinical suspicion. Conventional diagnosis is still largely used even though limitations are well known. Isolating the fungus is time consuming and requires manipulation in BSL3 facilities, while direct visualization and histopathology techniques show low sensitivity and need skilled personnel. New approaches based on the detection of antibodies and antigens have been developed and commercialized last years. Although sensitivity and specificity of these methods is variable, antigen detection has been recently listed as an essential diagnostic test for AIDS patients due to its excellent performance. DNA detection methods are recognized as promising tools but there is still a lack of consensus among laboratories and there are not commercial tests available. Not all methods are widely available, thus most laboratories combine classical and other tests in order to overcome aforementioned limitations. In this chapter, we review the diagnostic pipeline currently available for the diagnosis of histoplasmosis in microbiological laboratories, from conventional to new developed tests. Most recent approaches are introduced and future perspectives are discussed.

Keywords: histoplasmosis, diagnosis, culture, histopathology, PCR, antigen, antibody

1. Introduction

Histoplasmosis is caused by the thermally dimorphic fungi *Histoplasma capsulatum* and encompasses a broad variety of clinical presentations ranging from asymptomatic infections to subacute, acute and chronic pulmonary infections [1]. In immunosuppressed patients, especially in HIV positive population, it causes a progressive disseminated disease [2]. Mortality rates in AIDS population have been reported as 30–50% when treated, and 100% in absence of treatment [3]. Although this fungus has a cosmopolitan distribution, there are some areas of high endemicity as Ohio and Mississippi basins in North America, several countries from Central and South America and different regions in the African continent [4–6]. Areas of medium-high endemicity have been reported in China and some sporadic cases have been described in other regions of Asia as North of India, Thailand and Philippines [7–10]. The rest of the world is considered as non-endemic regions and reported cases are described as imported by travelers or immigrants [11]. It has been estimated that about a half million of people acquire the infection per year and around 100,000 develop a disseminated disease [3]. Certain regions of Brazil and Venezuela have been considered hotspots of the disseminated form of the disease [12]. However, in other regions as the African continent the incidence is probably underestimated due to lack of studies [6]. Diagnosis of histoplasmosis is challenging in both endemic and non-endemic regions due to its similarity to other diseases as tuberculosis, usually the first clinical suspicion, and the limitations and low availability of diagnostic tools. Consequently, many efforts have been recently made with the aim of improving diagnosis and combat histoplasmosis [3]. In this chapter, we describe the conventional methods used to diagnose histoplasmosis coupled with an update about the new tests available. The advantages and limitations of each method are detailed as well as their usefulness in the diagnosis regarding the diverse clinical presentations of the disease and their availability in the different regions. The need of continuous work on the development of new methods to achieve an early diagnosis and reduce histoplasmosis morbidity and mortality is also underlined.

2. Conventional diagnostic methods

Conventional diagnostic methods are still widely used for the diagnosis of histoplasmosis. The definite diagnosis is based on the isolation of the fungus in culture or the visualization of intracellular yeasts in tissues or other clinical samples. Thus, despite its known limitations, these methods are very useful and continue to be used in many laboratories, especially in low-resources settings.

2.1 Culture

The isolation of *H. capsulatum* in culture is the gold standard for the diagnosis of histoplasmosis. The recovery of the fungus by culture from clinical samples (blood culture, bronchoalveolar lavage fluid, etc.) is recognized as the criteria for the definition of proven histoplasmosis according to the consensus definitions of the European Organization for Research and Treatment of Cancer and the Mycoses Study Group Education and Research Consortium (EORTC-MSGERC) [13].

H. capsulatum is a so-called fastidious fungus since it can take up to 4 weeks to grow and requires Biosafety level 3 (BSL-3) containment measures [2]. At 25–30°C, it grows as a white and cottony mycelium that evolves to brown, representing the invasive form of the disease. This mycelial form is the most dangerous, as spores could be inhaled causing infection. Some laboratory-acquired infections have been reported by culture manipulation [14]. Microscopically the mycelial form produces the typical tuberculate macroconidia, which are easily identified (**Figure 1A**). However, other species as *Sepedonium* spp., an environmental organism that is usually considered as a laboratory contaminant, produce similar structures. At 37°C (human body temperature), there is a conversion from the mycelial phase to the yeast form, which is the pathogenic form of the disease. These yeasts are easily recognized by their thick wall and ovoid form with a narrow base at the smaller end (**Figure 1B**).

The sensitivity of cultures depends on the clinical status of the patient and the origin of the sample. Cultures are negative in most cases of asymptomatic and mild disease, however they are useful in disseminated and chronic pulmonary histoplasmosis, although their sensitivity varies from 50 to 85% [2, 15].

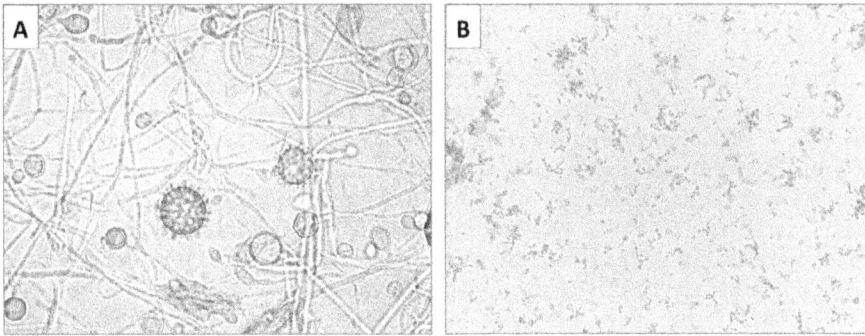

Figure 1.
Photomicrograph of lactophenol cotton blue stains of both filamentous and yeast forms of H. capsulatum.
(A) Culture at 30°C on potato dextrose agar (PDA) showing tuberculate macroconidia (63× magnification).
(B) Culture at 37°C on ML-GEMA medium showing yeasts (20× magnification). Both images belong to the
image library of the mycology reference laboratory (National Centre of Microbiology, Instituto de Salud
Carlos III, Madrid, Spain).

The main limitation of cultures is the long turnaround time needed to reach a definite diagnosis. Moreover, the microscopical observation of the grown fungus requires further confirmation by other methods. Molecular identification by sequencing the internal transcribed spacer (ITS) region of ribosomal DNA is a powerful tool to confirm the presence of *H. capsulatum*, but extends the time response for the diagnosis even more. Alternatively, single-stranded DNA probes could also be used to detect the fungus in cultures (AccuProbe, Hologic, CA, USA), however the procedure is technically complex and time consuming [16]. In last years, matrix-assisted laser desorption/ionization-time of flight mass spectrometry (MALDI-ToF MS) has started to be developed for the identification of *H. capsulatum* strains [17–19]. Although reports are still scarce, results in this area are promising since the system is able for recognizing different varieties (var. *capsulatum*, var. *duboisii*) and forms of the pathogen (yeast and mold), thus reducing response time and decreasing the risk of culture manipulation [19].

Since aforementioned limitations make culture useless for an early diagnosis of histoplasmosis, a great effort has been made for developing alternative diagnostic methods that could be used alone or in combination with cultures.

2.2 Histopathology and direct visualization

Direct examination of clinical samples or performing histopathological studies on tissues to detect yeast after staining with Gomori methenamine silver (GMS) or periodic acid-Schiff (PAS), are techniques largely used for the diagnosis of histoplasmosis. *H. capsulatum* could appear as a 2- to 4-μm (var. *capsulatum*) or 8- to 15-μm (var. *duboisii*) oval yeast. As yeasts are phagocytosed by macrophages, they could be found forming clusters, which can help the diagnosis. However, several fungi can be misled with *H. capsulatum* such as, among others, the small variant of *Blastomyces dermatitidis*, endospores of *Coccidioides* spp., *Candida glabrata* as well as the causal agents of leishmaniasis, toxoplasmosis, and Chagas' disease [20]. The higher sensitivity could be obtained in respiratory specimens or bone marrow biopsy in patients with disseminated histoplasmosis [21]. However, the low specificity and the need of skilled personnel to achieve a presumptive diagnosis are the main limitations of this technique.

3. Antigen detection

The detection of *H. capsulatum* antigens in clinical samples represented a breakthrough in the early diagnosis of histoplasmosis and has been included in the EORTC/MSG criteria for diagnosis of IFIs for almost 20 years [13, 22, 23]. The *H. capsulatum* polysaccharide antigen can be detected in both serum and urine samples with similar diagnostic value and has been recently listed as an essential diagnostic test for advanced AIDS patients [24, 25]. Two assays based on enzyme linked immunosorbent assay (ELISA) have been commercialized with good diagnostic performances (**Table 1**) although their availability is limited.

MiraVista's test presents great efficiency in serum and urine samples from patients with disseminated infection, but it is reduced in patients with pulmonary forms of the disease [26], in which BALF samples are more suitable for diagnosis [28]. This test is only performed in MVista's facilities then is not accessible out of USA limiting their use. On the other hand, IMMY has recently released an *Histoplasma* GM ELISA test which shows great performance and reproducibility, but has only be tested in urine samples [27]. Despite the high degree of cross-reaction with other fungi, antigen detection assays are widely used to diagnose histoplasmosis and some reports indicate its capacity to monitor treatment response [29, 30]. Nevertheless, their use is restricted mainly to developed endemic areas but it is rarely used in non-endemic regions, probably due to its low cost-effectiveness out of endemic regions [24, 31].

In last years, point-of-care (POC) testing has been emerged as a new diagnostic methodology and immuno-chromatographic assays performed in lateral-flow devices (LFD) are good examples. These "pregnancy tests-like" assays are easy to use, have low turnaround time (less than an hour) and require minimal laboratory equipment which facilitate its implementation in low- and middle-income countries [32, 33]. This technology was first developed for *Aspergillus* GM detection with great results and MVista has recently released a similar test consisting of a dipstick sandwich immunochromatographic assay based on the recognition of *H. capsulatum* GM antigen. Although it has only been tested in serum samples from AIDS patients, its diagnostic performance was very promising (sensitivity of 96%, specificity

Test[a]	Samples	Methodology	Turnaround time	Sensitivity/ specificity	Limitations
MV	Serum, plasma, urine, CSF, BALF, other body fluids	ELISA	Urine, BAL: <24 h Serum, plasma, CSF: 24 h	[b]DH: 92% APH: 83% SAPH: 30% CPH: 88%	• Cross-reactivity with other fungi • Samples are required to be shipped to the company's facilities
IMMY	Urine	ELISA	<2:15H	[c]95-98%/97-98%	• Cross-reactivity with other fungi

[a]MV: Histoplasma *Quantitative EIA test (MiraVista Diagnostics, Indianapolis, IN, USA); IMMY: CLARUS* Histoplasma *GM EIA kit (IMMY, Norman, OK, USA).*
[b]*DH [26].*
[c]*In 95-98% [27].*
ELISA: enzyme-linked immunosorbent assay; CSF: cerebrospinal fluid; BALF: bronchoalveolar lavage fluid; DH: disseminated histoplasmosis; APH: acute pulmonary histoplasmosis; SAPH: sub-acute pulmonary histoplasmosis; CPH: chronic pulmonary histoplamosis; GM: galactomannan.

Table 1.
Main characteristics and diagnostic performance of commercial assays for detecting H. capsulatum *antigens.*

of 90%) [34]. However, false positive and negative results still occurred due to cross-reactivity with other endemic fungi and antibiotic treatment, respectively, and a pre-treatment step was required extending turnaround times. Currently, a new LFD test is being developed and validated by using urine samples [35].

4. Antibody detection

The main advantages of antibody detection tests are the requirement of minimally invasive samples and the achievement of results when culture is still negative reducing the need of handling potentially infectious fungi [36]. Serological techniques such as complement fixation or immunodiffusion are useful when testing samples from travelers coming from endemic regions for the first time. Both techniques are commercially available (Immuno Mycologics, Norman, OK, USA) and the sensitivity of these tests in acute and subacute pulmonary histoplasmosis has been reported as 95% [37]. However, sensitivity is very limited in immunosuppressed patients due to low or absent antibody titers. A recent meta-analysis described sensitivity and specificity values of 58% and 100%, respectively, in samples from HIV patients [38]. Finally, since seropositivity remains long time after disease, interpretation of serological results could be challenging [39, 40]. Despite the limitations previously described, antibody detection tests are still considered as valuable diagnostic tools and have been demonstrated to improve diagnostic yield when combined with other diagnostic methods [41, 42].

5. DNA based detection methods

PCR methods based on the detection of fungal DNA directly from clinical samples are currently implemented in the routine of several laboratories for the diagnosis of main fungal infections, but there are considerably fewer PCR tests for the diagnosis of histoplasmosis. Their advantages rely on their simplicity, high specificity and short turnaround time with the bonus that real-time PCR (qPCR) formats allow for determining the fungal burden in patients by using non-specific DNA-binding dyes or fluorescently labeled probes [36, 43]. However, this technique also has some limitations as the moderate amount of DNA in low invasive samples, the lack of standardization and the low availability of widely validated commercial systems [44, 45]. Recently, PCR based methods have been included in the EORTC/MSG criteria for the diagnosis of some fungal infections such as invasive aspergillosis or candidiasis but not for endemic mycoses [13].

The majority of PCR tests for the diagnosis of histoplasmosis have been developed in house and none of them has been commercialized. They have been recently reviewed in several reports with different purposes [31, 38, 46]. Most developed methods targeted specific multicopy regions of the ribosomal DNA or the single-copy Hcp100 gene and were performed by using conventional, nested or qPCR formats. The sensitivity and specificity of these assays depends on the type of sample analyzed, the clinical characteristics of patients and the PCR format used for DNA detection. These tests showed an excellent analytical performance (overall sensitivity of 95% and specificity of 99%) when testing samples of HIV patients [38], but sensitivity decreased when testing blood and serum samples from immunocompetent patients [31, 46]. Panfungal or broad-range PCRs are used when there is not a clear suspicion of the fungus involved in the infection, since universal primers are used to detect any fungal DNA in the clinical sample. Although studies are scarce, several reports achieved the detection of

H. capsulatum DNA in clinical samples by using this technique, which could be especially useful in non-endemic regions [47–51].

Non-PCR based methods are also able to amplify and detect *H. capsulatum* DNA from clinical samples. Loop-mediated isothermal amplification (LAMP) rests on the use of a DNA polymerase with high displacement strand activity and a set of specifically designed primers to amplify targeted DNA [52]. Some reports described the implementation of this technique for the molecular diagnosis of histoplasmosis showing great results [53, 54]. The high efficiency, sensitivity, specificity and cost-effectiveness of these assays make them good candidates to be implemented in the diagnostic routine of resource-limited laboratories.

6. Conclusions and future perspectives

Early diagnosis of histoplasmosis is essential to establish a suitable antifungal therapy, which results in the reduction of mortality rates [55, 56]. This becomes especially important in certain hyper-endemic regions since they usually are disfavored areas where patients develop the disease in its disseminated form. While culture and histopathological examination are considered the gold standards methods for histoplasmosis diagnosis, these techniques show moderate sensitivity. In addition, culture is time consuming, requiring handling fungi in BSL-3 facilities. New approaches as MALDI-ToF MS technology allow for a rapid identification, but studies are still scarce. Antibody and antigen detection are useful tools for an early detection of the pathogen in low invasive clinical samples such as serum and urine. Despite limitations concerning sensitivity in certain populations and specificity have been widely reported, *H. capsulatum* antigen detection has been recently included in the second edition of the list of essential in vitro diagnostics (https://www.who.int/medical_devices/diagnostics/selection_in-vitro/selection_in-vitro-meetings/sage-ivd2nd-meeting/190318-2ndEditionofEDL-open-session.pdf?ua=1). Regarding molecular methods, in the last decade a great effort has been made on the development of PCR tests for the detection of *H. capsulatum* DNA in a broad spectrum of clinical samples showing excellent diagnostic performance. However, a consensus among laboratories about the best samples, targets and procedures is mandatory. Consequently, no commercial tests are available to date limiting the use of this technique. To date, only an inter-laboratory study focused on molecular techniques for the diagnosis of histoplasmosis has been published [57]. In this work, authors concluded that qPCR targeting a multicopy genomic region was the best option for a suitable sensitivity. A European initiative is being launched to carry out multicenter studies in this regard.

All these problems have gained attention thanks to different initiatives coming from researchers from hyper-endemic regions [58] or international foundations as the Global Action Fund for Fungal Infections (GAFFI). As a result, proposals such as the Manaus declaration have been launched, specifically to get access to rapid testing for histoplasmosis in the Americas and Caribe until 2025 (https://www.gaffi.org/the-manaus-declaration-on-histoplasmosis-in-the-americas-and-carib-bean-100-by-2025/). However, in addition to these excellent initiatives further work is required to improve diagnosis. In this sense, novel techniques as next generation sequencing (NGS) have been found to be useful in the diagnosis of several infec-tions. Sequences obtained from clinical samples through NGS can be compared against reference databases enabling their identification to the genus and species level [59]. This technique has been used recently to identify *H. capsulatum* as the causal agent of a case of chronic meningitis [60] and for the differential diagnosis among histoplasmosis, leishmaniosis and talaromycosis [61]. Another approach

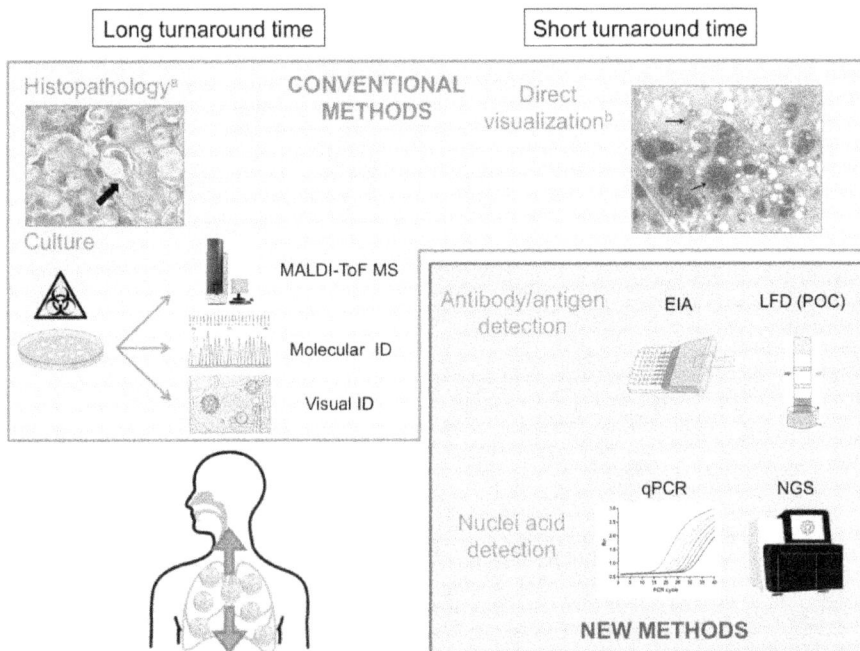

Figure 2.
Diagnostic pipeline currently available for the microbiological diagnosis of histoplasmosis. [a]Histopathological preparation showing a H. capsulatum *yeast budding [62]. [b]Direct visualization of fine needle aspiration cytology showing intra- and extracellular yeasts of* H. capsulatum *[63]. MALDI-ToF MS: matrix-assisted laser desorption/ionization-time of flight mass spectrometry; ID: identification; EIA: enzyme immunoassay; LFD: lateral flow device; POC: point of care; qPCR: quantitative PCR; NGS: next generation sequencing.*

in constant development is based on determining host and fungal biomarkers that could indicate the presence of *H. capsulatum* in human body fluids. Recent advances in antibody detection are related to the refinement of antibody detection platforms (*Histoplasma* antibody IgG IgM EIA, MiraVista Diagnostics), while most efforts in antigen detection are focused on improving diagnostic yields of POC methods [35].

In summary, the aim of this chapter was to summarize the diagnostic pipeline currently available for the diagnosis of histoplasmosis in microbiological laboratories (**Figure 2**). Although so much progress has been made in the area, much certainly remains to be done to improve the early diagnosis of histoplasmosis, allowing the establishment of a prompt antifungal therapy and consequently reducing morbidity and mortality rates of this infection.

Conflict of interest

The authors declare no conflict of interest.

Author details

María J. Buitrago[1*] and Clara Valero[1,2]

1 Reference Laboratory in Mycology, National Center for Microbiology, Instituto de Salud Carlos III, Madrid, Spain

2 School of Pharmaceutical Sciences of Ribeirão Preto, University of São Paulo, Ribeirão Preto, Brazil

*Address all correspondence to: buitrago@isciii.es

IntechOpen

References

[1] Kauffman CA. Histoplasmosis. Clinics in Chest Medicine. 2009;**30**(2):217-225. DOI: 10.1016/j. ccm.2009.02.002

[2] Wheat LJ, Azar MM, Bahr NC, Spec A, Relich RF, Hage C. Histoplasmosis. Infectious Disease Clinics of North America. 2016;**30**(1):207-227. DOI: 10.1016/j. idc.2015.10.009

[3] Bongomin F, Kwizera R, Denning DW. Getting histoplasmosis on the map of international recommendations for patients with advanced HIV disease. Journal of Fungi. 2019;**5**(3). DOI: 10.3390/jof5030080

[4] Benedict K, Mody RK. Epidemiology of histoplasmosis outbreaks, United States, 1938-2013. Emerging Infectious Diseases. 2016;**22**(3):370-378. DOI: 10.3201/eid2203.151117

[5] Colombo AL, Tobon A, Restrepo A, Queiroz-Telles F, Nucci M. Epidemiology of endemic systemic fungal infections in Latin America. Medical Mycology. 2011;**49**(8):785-798. DOI: 10.3109/13693786.2011.577821

[6] Oladele RO, Ayanlowo OO, Richardson MD, Denning DW. Histoplasmosis in Africa: An emerging or a neglected disease? PLoS Neglected Tropical Diseases. 2018;**12**(1):e0006046. DOI: 10.1371/journal.pntd.0006046

[7] Antinori S. *Histoplasma capsulatum*: More widespread than previously thought. The American Journal of Tropical Medicine and Hygiene. 2014;**90**(6):982-983. DOI: 10.4269/ajtmh.14-0175

[8] Bulmer AC, Bulmer GS. Incidence of histoplasmin hypersensitivity in the Philippines. Mycopathologia. 2001;**149**(2):69-71. DOI: 10.1023/a:1007277602576

[9] Kathuria S, Capoor MR, Yadav S, Singh A, Ramesh V. Disseminated histoplasmosis in an apparentlyimmunocompetentindividual from North India: A case report and review. Medical Mycology. 2013;**51**(7):774-778. DOI: 10.3109/13693786.2013.777166

[10] Rangwala F, Putcharoen O, Bowonwatanuwong C, Edwards-Jackson N, Kramomthong S, Kim JH, et al. Histoplasmosis and penicilliosis among HIV-infected Thai patients: A retrospective review. The Southeast Asian Journal of Tropical Medicine and Public Health. 2012;**43**(2):436-441

[11] Molina-Morant D, Sanchez-Montalva A, Salvador F, Sao-Aviles A, Molina I. Imported endemic mycoses in Spain: Evolution of hospitalized cases, clinical characteristics and correlation with migratory movements, 1997-2014. PLoS Neglected Tropical Diseases. 2018;**12**(2):e0006245. DOI: 10.1371/journal.pntd.0006245

[12] Denning DW. Minimizing fungal disease deaths will allow the UNAIDS target of reducing annual AIDS deaths below 500,000 by 2020 to be realized. Philosophical Transactions of the Royal Society of London Series B, Biological Sciences. 2016;**371**(1709). DOI: 10.1098/rstb.2015.0468

[13] Donnelly JP, Chen SC, Kauffman CA, Steinbach WJ, Baddley JW, Verweij PE, et al. Revision and update of the consensus definitions of invasive fungal disease from the European Organization for Research and Treatment of Cancer and the Mycoses Study Group Education and Research Consortium. Clinical Infectious Diseases. 2019;ciz1008 (online ahead of print). DOI: 10.1093/cid/ciz1008

[14] Fleming DO, Hunt DL. Biological Safety, Principles and Practices. 4th ed.

Washington: ASM Press; 2006. DOI: 10.1590/S0036-46652001000600013

[15] Azar MM, Hage CA. Laboratory diagnostics for histoplasmosis. Journal of Clinical Microbiology. 2017;**55**(6):1612-1620. DOI: 10.1128/JCM.02430-16

[16] Gómez BL. Molecular diagnosis of endemic and invasive mycoses: Advances and challenges. Revista Iberoamericana de Micología. 2014;**31**(1):35-41. DOI: 10.1016/j.riam.2013.09.009

[17] Lau AF, Drake SK, Calhoun LB, Henderson CM, Zelazny AM. Development of a clinically comprehensive database and a simple procedure for identification of molds from solid media by matrix-assisted laser desorption ionization-time of flight mass spectrometry. Journal of Clinical Microbiology. 2013;**51**(3):828-834. DOI: 10.1128/JCM.02852-12

[18] Rychert J, Slechta ES, Barker AP, Miranda E, Babady NE, Tang YW, et al. Multicenter evaluation of the Vitek MS v3.0 system for the identification of filamentous fungi. Journal of Clinical Microbiology. 2018;**56**(2):e01353-17. DOI: 10.1128/JCM.01353-17

[19] Valero C, Buitrago MJ, Gago S, Quiles-Melero I, García-Rodríguez J. A matrix-assisted laser desorption/ionization time of flight mass spectrometry reference database for the identification of *Histoplasma capsulatum*. Medical Mycology. 2018;**56**(3):307-314. DOI: 10.1093/mmy/myx047

[20] Guarner J, Brandt ME. Histopathologic diagnosis of fungal infections in the 21st century. Clinical Microbiology Reviews. 2011;**24**(2):247-280. DOI: 10.1128/CMR.00053-10

[21] Kauffman CA. Histoplasmosis: A clinical and laboratory update. Clinical Microbiology Reviews.

2007;**20**(1):115-132. DOI: 10.1128/CMR.00027-06

[22] Ascioglu S, Rex JH, de Pauw B, Bennett JE, Bille J, Crokaert F, et al. Defining opportunistic invasive fungal infections in immunocompromised patients with cancer and hematopoietic stem cell transplants: An international consensus. Clinical Infectious Diseases. 2002;**34**(1):7-14. DOI: 10.1086/323335

[23] De Pauw B, Walsh TJ, Donnelly JP, Stevens DA, Edwards JE, Calandra T, et al. Revised definitions of invasive fungal disease from the European Organization for Research and Treatment of Cancer/invasive fungal infections cooperative group and the National Institute of Allergy and Infectious Diseases Mycoses Study Group (EORTC/MSG) Consensus Group. Clinical Infectious Diseases. 2008;**46**(12):1813-1821. DOI: 10.1086/588660

[24] Bongomin F, Govender NP, Chakrabarti A, Robert-Gangneux F, Boulware DR, Zafar A, et al. Essential *in vitro* diagnostics for advanced HIV and serious fungal diseases: International experts' consensus recommendations. European Journal of Clinical Microbiology & Infectious Diseases. 2019;**38**(9):1581-1584. DOI: 10.1007/s10096-019-03600-4

[25] Fandiño-Devia E, Rodríguez-Echeverri C, Cardona-Arias J, González A. Antigen detection in the diagnosis of histoplasmosis: A meta-analysis of diagnostic performance. Mycopathologia. 2016;**181**(3-4):197-205. DOI: 10.1007/s11046-015-9965-3

[26] Hage CA, Azar MM, Bahr N, Loyd J, Wheat LJ. Histoplasmosis: Up-to-date evidence-based approach to diagnosis and management. Seminars in Respiratory and Critical Care Medicine. 2015;**36**(5):729-745. DOI: 10.1055/s-0035-1562899

[27] Cáceres DH, Samayoa BE, Medina NG, Tobon AM, Guzmán BJ,

Mercado D, et al. Multicenter validation of commercial antigenuria reagents to diagnose progressive disseminated histoplasmosis in people living with HIV/AIDS in two Latin American countries. Journal of Clinical Microbiology. 2018;**56**(6). DOI: 10.1128/JCM.01959-17

[28] Hage CA, Wheat LJ. Diagnosis of pulmonary histoplasmosis using antigen detection in the bronchoalveolar lavage. Expert Review of Respiratory Medicine. 2010;**4**(4):427-429. DOI: 10.1586/ers.10.36

[29] Cáceres DH, Scheel CM, Tobon AM, Ahlquist Cleveland A, Restrepo A, Brandt ME, et al. Validation of an enzyme-linked immunosorbent assay that detects *Histoplasma capsulatum* antigenuria in Colombian patients with AIDS for diagnosis and follow-up during therapy. Clinical and Vaccine Immunology. 2014;**21**(9):1364-1368. DOI: 10.1128/CVI.00101-14

[30] Hage CA, Kirsch EJ, Stump TE, Kauffman CA, Goldman M, Connolly P, et al. *Histoplasma* antigen clearance during treatment of histoplasmosis in patients with AIDS determined by a quantitative antigen enzyme immunoassay. Clinical and Vaccine Immunology. 2011;**18**(4):661-666. DOI: 10.1128/CVI.00389-10

[31] Buitrago MJ, Martin-Gomez MT. Timely diagnosis of histoplasmosis in non-endemic countries: A laboratory challenge. Frontiers in Microbiology. 2020;**11**:467. DOI: 10.3389/fmicb.2020.00467

[32] Kozel TR, Burnham-Marusich AR. Point-of-care testing for infectious diseases: Past, present, and future. Journal of Clinical Microbiology. 2017;**55**(8):2313-2320. DOI: 10.1128/JCM.00476-17

[33] Prattes J, Heldt S, Eigl S, Hoenigl M. Point of care testing for the diagnosis of fungal infections: Are we there yet? Current Fungal Infection Reports. 2016;**10**:43-50. DOI: 10.1007/s12281-016-0254-5

[34] Cáceres DH, Gómez BL, Tobon AM, Chiller TM, Lindsley MD. Evaluation of a *Histoplasma* antigen lateral flow assay for the rapid diagnosis of progressive disseminated histoplasmosis in Colombian patients with AIDS. Mycoses. 2020;**63**(2):139-144. DOI: 10.1111/myc.13023

[35] Myint T, Leedy N, Villacorta Cari E, Wheat LJ. HIV-associated histoplasmosis: Current perspectives. HIV/AIDS. 2020;**12**:113-125. DOI: 10.2147/HIV.S185631

[36] Kozel TR, Wickes B. Fungal diagnostics. Cold Spring Harbor Perspectives in Medicine. 2014;**4**(4):a019299. DOI: 10.1101/cshperspect.a019299

[37] Hage CA, Knox KS, Wheat LJ. Endemic mycoses: Overlooked causes of community acquired pneumonia. Respiratory Medicine. 2012;**106**(6):769-776. DOI: 10.1016/j.rmed.2012.02.004

[38] Cáceres DH, Knuth M, Derado G, Lindsley MD. Diagnosis of progressive disseminated histoplasmosis in advanced HIV: A meta-analysis of assay analytical performance. Journal of Fungi. 2019;**5**(3). DOI: 10.3390/jof5030076

[39] Ramanan P, Wengenack NL, Theel ES. Laboratory diagnostics for fungal infections: A review of current and future diagnostic assays. Clinics in Chest Medicine. 2017;**38**(3):535-554. DOI: 10.1016/j.ccm.2017.04.013

[40] Richardson M, Page I. Role of serological tests in the diagnosis of mold infections. Current Fungal Infection Reports. 2018;**12**(3):127-136. DOI: 10.1007/s12281-018-0321-1

[41] Bloch KC, Myint T, Raymond-Guillen L, Hage CA, Davis TE, Wright PW, et al. Improvement in diagnosis of *Histoplasma* meningitis by combined testing for *Histoplasma* antigen and immunoglobulin G and immunoglobulin M anti-*Histoplasma* antibody in cerebrospinal fluid. Clinical Infectious Diseases. 2018;**66**(1):89-94. DOI: 10.1093/cid/cix706

[42] Richer SM, Smedema ML, Durkin MM, Herman KM, Hage CA, Fuller D, et al. Improved diagnosis of acute pulmonary histoplasmosis by combining antigen and antibody detection. Clinical Infectious Diseases. 2016;**62**(7):896-902. DOI: 10.1093/cid/ciw007

[43] Arvanitis M, Anagnostou T, Fuchs BB, Caliendo AM, Mylonakis E. Molecular and nonmolecular diagnostic methods for invasive fungal infections. Clinical Microbiology Reviews. 2014;**27**(3):490-526. DOI: 10.1128/CMR.00091-13

[44] Alanio A, Bretagne S. Performance evaluation of multiplex PCR including *Aspergillus*-not so simple! Medical Mycology. 2017;**55**(1):56-62. DOI: 10.1093/mmy/myw080

[45] Khot PD, Fredricks DN. PCR-based diagnosis of human fungal infections. Expert Review of Anti-Infective Therapy. 2009;7(10):1201-1221. DOI: 10.1586/eri.09.104

[46] Vasconcellos I, Dalla Lana DF, Pasqualotto AC. The role of molecular tests in the diagnosis of disseminated histoplasmosis. Journal of Fungi. 2019;**6**(1). DOI: 10.3390/jof6010001

[47] Ala-Houhala M, Koukila-Kahkola P, Antikainen J, Valve J, Kirveskari J, Anttila VJ. Clinical use of fungal PCR from deep tissue samples in the diagnosis of invasive fungal diseases: A retrospective observational study. Clinical Microbiology and Infection.

2018;**24**(3):301-305. DOI: 10.1016/j.cmi.2017.08.017

[48] Buitrago MJ, Bernal-Martínez L, Castelli MV, Rodríguez-Tudela JL, Cuenca-Estrella M. Performance of panfungal and specific PCR based procedures for etiological diagnosis of invasive fungal diseases on tissue biopsy specimens with proven infection: A 7-year retrospective analysis from a reference laboratory. Journal of Clinical Microbiology. 2014;**52**(5):1737-1740. DOI: 10.1128/JCM.00328-14

[49] Gómez CA, Budvytiene I, Zemek AJ, Banaei N. Performance of targeted fungal sequencing for culture-independent diagnosis of invasive fungal disease. Clinical Infectious Diseases. 2017;**65**(12):2035-2041. DOI: 10.1093/cid/cix728

[50] Lindner AK, Rickerts V, Kurth F, Wilmes D, Richter J. Chronic oral ulceration and lip swelling after a long term stay in Guatemala: A diagnostic challenge. Travel Medicine and Infectious Disease. 2018;**23**:103-104. DOI: 10.1016/j.tmaid.2018.04.009

[51] Valero C, de la Cruz-Villar L, Zaragoza Ó, Buitrago MJ. New panfungal real-time PCR assay for diagnosis of invasive fungal infections. Journal of Clinical microbiology. 2016;**54**(12):2910-2918. DOI: 10.1128/JCM.01580-16

[52] Wong YP, Othman S, Lau YL, Radu S, Chee HY. Loop-mediated isothermal amplification (LAMP): A versatile technique for detection of microorganisms. Journal of Applied Microbiology. 2018;**124**(3):626-643. DOI: 10.1111/jam.13647

[53] Scheel CM, Zhou Y, Theodoro RC, Abrams B, Balajee SA, Litvintseva AP. Development of a loop-mediated isothermal amplification method for detection of *Histoplasma capsulatum* DNA in clinical samples. Journal of

Clinical Microbiology. 2014;**52**(2):483-488. DOI: 10.1128/JCM.02739-13

[54] Zatti MDS, Arantes TD, Fernandes JAL, Bay MB, Milan EP, Naliato GFS, et al. Loop-mediated isothermal amplification and nested PCR of the internal transcribed spacer (ITS) for *Histoplasma capsulatum* detection. PLoS Neglected Tropical Diseases. 2019;**13**(8):e0007692. DOI: 10.1371/journal.pntd.0007692

[55] Adenis AA, Aznar C, Couppie P. Histoplasmosis in HIV-infected patients: A review of new developments and remaining gaps. Current Tropical Medicine Reports. 2014;**1**:119-128. DOI: 10.1007/s40475-014-0017-8

[56] Scheel CM, Gómez BL. Diagnostic methods for histoplasmosis: Focus on endemic countries with variable infrastructure levels. Current Tropical Medicine Reports. 2014;**1**(2):129-137. DOI: 10.1007/s40475-014-0020-0

[57] Buitrago MJ, Canteros CE, Frías De León G, González Á, Marques-Evangelista De Oliveira M, Muñoz CO, et al. Comparison of PCR protocols for detecting *Histoplasma capsulatum* DNA through a multicenter study. Revista Iberoamericana de Micología. 2013;**30**(4):256-260. DOI: 10.1016/j.riam.2013.03.004

[58] Nacher M, Adenis A, Mc Donald S, Do Socorro Mendonca Gomes M, Singh S, Lopes Lima I, et al. Disseminated histoplasmosis in HIV-infected patients in South America: A neglected killer continues on its rampage. PLoS Neglected Tropical Disease. 2013;**7**, **11**:e2319. DOI: 10.1371/journal.pntd.0002319

[59] Kidd SE, Chen SC, Meyer W, Halliday CL. A new age in molecular diagnostics for invasive fungal disease: Are we ready? Frontiers in Microbiology. 2019;**10**:2903. DOI: 10.3389/fmicb.2019.02903

[60] Wilson MR, O'Donovan BD, Gelfand JM, Sample HA, Chow FC, Betjemann JP, et al. Chronic meningitis investigated via metagenomic next-generation sequencing. JAMA Neurology. 2018;**75**(8):947-955. DOI: 10.1001/jamaneurol.2018.0463

[61] Zhang HC, Zhang QR, Ai JW, Cui P, Wu HL, Zhang WH, et al. The role of bone marrow metagenomics next-generation sequencing to differential diagnosis among visceral leishmaniasis, histoplasmosis, and talaromycosis marneffei. International Journal of Laboratory Hematology. 2020;**42**(2):e52-e54. DOI: 10.1111/ijlh.13103

[62] Pakasa N, Biber A, Nsiangana S, Imposo D, Sumaili E, Muhindo H, et al. African histoplasmosis in HIV-negative patients, Kimpese, Democratic Republic of the Congo. Emerging Infectious Diseases. 2018;**24**(11):2068-2070. DOI: 10.3201/eid2411.180236

[63] Mahajan VK, Raina RK, Singh S, Rashpa RS, Sood A, Chauhan PS, et al. Case report: Histoplasmosis in Himachal Pradesh (India): An emerging endemic focus. The American Journal of Tropical Medicine and Hygiene. 2017;**97**(6):1749-1756. DOI: 10.4269/ajtmh.17-0432

Section 4

Treatment

Chapter 5

Treatment of Histoplasmosis

Felix Bongomin, Richard Kwizera, Joseph Baruch Baluku,
Lucy Grace Asio and Akaninyene A. Otu

Abstract

Histoplasmosis, caused by the thermally dimorphic fungus *Histoplasma capsulatum*, is an uncommon multisystem disease with a global distribution. The spectrum of clinical manifestations ranges from an asymptomatic or minimally symptomatic acute pulmonary disease following inhalation of a large inoculum of *Histoplasma* microconidia to chronic pulmonary disease in patients with underlying structural lung disease. It also extends to acute progressive disseminated disease in patients with severe immunodeficiency. Generally, antifungal therapy is indicated for patients with progressive acute pulmonary histoplasmosis, chronic pulmonary histoplasmosis and acute progressive disseminated histoplasmosis. In immunocompetent patients, acute pulmonary histoplasmosis may be a self-limiting disease without the need for systemic antifungal therapy. Oral triazole antifungal drugs alone are recommended for less severe disease. However, moderate-to-severe acute pulmonary histoplasmosis requires intravenous amphotericin B therapy for at least 1–2 weeks followed by oral itraconazole for at least 12 weeks. For acute progressive disseminated histoplasmosis, intravenous amphotericin B therapy is given for at least 2 weeks (4–6 weeks if meningeal involvement) or until a patient can tolerate oral therapy, followed by oral itraconazole (or an alternative triazole) for at least 12 months. Chronic cavitary pulmonary histoplasmosis is treated with oral itraconazole for 1–2 years. There is insufficient evidence to support the use of isavuconazole or the echinocandins for the treatment of histoplasmosis.

Keywords: *Histoplasma capsulatum*, histoplasmosis, itraconazole, amphotericin B, HIV

1. Introduction

Histoplasmosis is an uncommon endemic mycosis caused by the fungus *Histoplasma capsulatum* that usually causes an asymptomatic infection but occasionally results in severe multisystem disease [1, 2]. Two main varieties of the saprophytic, thermally dimorphic fungus of the genus *Histoplasma* affect humans; *Histoplasma capsulatum var. capsulatum* and *Histoplasma capsulatum var. duboisii* [3–5]. Histoplasmosis affects over 10,000 people globally; it is neglected, worryingly under-diagnosed, and often misdiagnosed as cancer or tuberculosis with fatal consequences [6–8]. The spectrum of the clinical manifestation of histoplasmosis is very broad, ranging from an asymptomatic or minimally symptomatic acute pulmonary disease following inhalation of a large inoculum of *Histoplasma* microconidia to chronic pulmonary disease in patients with underlying structural lung disease, to acute progressive disseminated disease in patients with severe immunodeficiency [9–13]. In immunocompetent patients, acute histoplasmosis is typically a self-limiting disease with no need for antifungal therapy [14]. Pneumonia remains the most common disease presentation but extrapulmonary dissemination can occur, especially in immunocompromised patients [12]. A definite diagnosis of histoplasmosis is based on the isolation of the organisms in fungal culture [15]. Rapid detection of the *H. capsulatum* polysaccharide antigen using enzyme immunoassay (EIA) in urine, blood or bronchoalveolar lavage fluid is also available and very useful especially among immunocompromised patients with disseminated or acute pulmonary disease [13, 16]. Serologic testing for antibodies can be achieved by EIA, immunodiffusion, and complement fixation [13, 16, 17]. These antibody tests may be falsely negative in immunosuppressed patients and are most valuable when combined with a compatible clinical presentation and epidemiologic risk factors.

This chapter provides an overview of the currently available treatment options for the different manifestations of histoplasmosis.

2. Antifungal agents used in the treatment of histoplasmosis

Histoplasmosis is primarily treated with 2 distinct classes of antifungal agents: The triazoles and the polyenes. Data is lacking on the use of the echinocandins for the treatment of histoplasmosis.

2.1 Triazole

The triazole class of antifungals examples of which includes drug like fluconazole, itraconazole, voriconazole, posaconazole and isavuconazole [18, 19]. Of these, itraconazole is the drug of choice for the treatment of the various forms of histoplasmosis as a sole therapy or as a step-down therapy following amphotericin B infusion [13, 14, 20].

Triazole antifungals inhibit the cytochrome P450-dependent enzyme 14-alpha-lanosterol demethylase (CYP51) encoded by the *ERG11* gene that converts lanosterol to ergosterol in the cell membrane, inhibiting fungal growth and replication (fungistatic) [18, 19]. Drug-drug and drug-food interactions, as well as side effects are major issues associated with itraconazole therapy. Common side effects of itraconazole include drug-induced hepatitis, gastrointestinal discomfort, heart failure, ankle edema, alopecia, erectile dysfunction, gynaecomastia, peripheral neuropathy, visual disturbance and headaches [21]. Itraconazole interacts with agents used in the treatment of HIV (especially, nevirapine) and tuberculosis (especially, rifampicin) leading to decreased or increased exposures to itraconazole and therefore increased risk of hepatotoxicity. With the exception of fluconazole, voriconazole and posaconazole are used as alternative agents for the treatment of histoplasmosis if there is a contraindication to the use of itraconazole [13, 14, 20]. However, to the best of our knowledge, there is no data to support the use of isavuconazole for the treatment of histoplasmosis.

2.2 Polyene

The polyene antibiotic, amphotericin B derived from the fermentation product of the filamentous bacteria, *Streptomyces nodosus* is a broad-spectrum antifungal agent administered as deoxycholate (conventional amphotericin B) or liposomal formulation [18, 19].

In its mechanism of action, amphotericin B preferentially binds ergosterol in the fungal cell membrane (and to a lesser extent, cholesterol in cell membrane of humans) to form channels through which small molecules leak from the inside of the fungal cell to the outside, resulting in death of the fungal cell (fungicidal) [18, 19].

Common side effects of amphotericin B include, acute infusion-related reactions characterised by nausea, vomiting, rigors, fever, hyper or hypotension, and hypoxia mainly driven by the effects of amphotericin B on pro-inflammatory cytokine production. Nephrotoxicity is another very important side effect of amphotericin B occurring in about 34–60% of patients. Blood disorders, especially anaemia and electrolyte disturbances, especially hypomagnesaemia and hypokalemia are common but can be part of the rare Fanconi syndrome. Other side effects include infusion site phlebitis, and acute kidney injury [21].

3. Overview of antifungal treatment of histoplasmosis

It is important to understand the indications and the choices of antifungal agents in the treatment of histoplasmosis. Manifestations of histoplasmosis that are a typically treated include moderate to severe acute pulmonary histoplasmosis, symptomatic chronic cavitary pulmonary histoplasmosis, acute progressive disseminated disease, and histoplasmosis in immunocompromised individuals [12, 13], (**Table 1**). Treatment is also indicated for complications of histoplasmosis such as mediastinal granulomas and adenitis [14], (**Table 1**). Itraconazole can be used for the treatment of symptomatic immunocompetent patients with indolent non-meningeal infection, including chronic cavitary pulmonary histoplasmosis [12, 13]. Itraconazole is also used as a step-down oral agent following initial treatment of severe disease with amphotericin B [12, 13]. Itraconazole is administered at a dose 200 mg 3 times daily for 3 days, as loading dose and then 200 mg once or twice daily, for maintenance therapy [12, 13]. Duration of itraconazole therapy depends on the histoplasmosis syndrome being managed (**Table 1**).

Amphotericin by intravenous infusion is the drug of choice for the initial treatment of fulminant or moderate to severe infections, followed by a course of oral. Following successful treatment, itraconazole can be used for secondary prophylaxis against relapse until immune reconstitution is realised [12, 13]. The deoxycholate formulation of amphotericin B is administered at a dose of 0.7–1.0 mg/kg daily by intravenous infusion, meanwhile the lipid formulation of amphotericin B can be administered at a higher dose of 3.0–5.0 mg/kg daily. Liposomal formulation is preferred to the deoxycholate due to its superior side effect profile, better response rate and survival benefit [14, 20].

3.1 Central nervous system histoplasmosis

There are no known prospective studies that have evaluated treatment of central nervous system (CNS) histoplasmosis. Treatment recommendations are guided by several case reports, retrospective case series and expert opinion [12, 13].

Liposomal amphotericin B achieves higher CNS concentrations than deoxycholate formulations and together with triazoles, is the recommended therapy for CNS histoplasmosis [22]. While the choice of the optimal triazole is in doubt, there is evidence from an animal model to suggest that fluconazole may be antagonistic when combined with amphotericin B [23]. Voriconazole could have a role among patients with good performance status as monotherapy or in combination with amphotericin B, but the evidence is limited and the occurrence of hepatotoxicity and hypersensitivity may limit its use [24–26]. One case series of 11 cases reported a morbidity free survival of 54.5% when patients were treated with intravenous amphotericin B deoxycholate for 8 weeks followed by maintenance therapy with fluconazole or itraconazole for 12–18 months [27].

Histoplasmosis syndrome or complication	Risk factor	Clinical time-course	Indication for treatment	Treatment		Antifungal therapy duration
Acute progressive disseminated histoplasmosis	Immunosuppression such as advanced HIV disease	1–2 weeks	Always	Mild disease	Itraconazole	12 months followed by maintenance antifungal suppression until immune recovery
				Moderate to severe disease	Amphotericin B for 1–2 weeks in non-meningeal and 4–6 weeks in meningeal disease followed by itraconazole as step-down therapy	
Acute pulmonary histoplasmosis	High inoculum exposure to Histoplasma conidia	1–2 weeks	Moderate or severe disease or immunosuppressed patient	Mild disease	Itraconazole	12 weeks
				Severe disease	Amphotericin B for 1–2 weeks followed by itraconazole as step-down therapy	
Subacute pulmonary histoplasmosis	Low inoculum exposure to Histoplasma conidia	Weeks to months	If symptoms last >1 months or immunosuppressed patient	Itraconazole		6–12 weeks
Chronic cavitary pulmonary histoplasmosis	Chronic obstructive pulmonary disease and other lung diseases Smoking	Months to years	Always	Itraconazole		1–2 years and until radiologic resolution or stabilisation
Mediastinal adenitis	Reactive and enlarged mediastinal lymph nodes	Early complication	If compressive symptoms present or adenitis last >1 months	Itraconazole and steroids		6–12 weeks
Mediastinal granuloma	Coalesced necrotic mediastinal lymph nodes	Early or late complication	If compressive symptoms present	Surgery and itraconazole		6–12 weeks
Mediastinal fibrosis	Fibrosis of mediastinal structures	Late complication	If compressive symptoms present	Stenting, arterial embolization or surgery		Not applicable

Table 1.
Treatment of histoplasmosis syndromes and their complications [13, 14].

The Infectious Diseases Society of America (IDSA) recommends treating CNS disease with liposomal amphotericin B (3.0–5.0 mg/kg daily for a total of 175 mg/kg given over 4–6 weeks), followed by a maintenance phase with itraconazole for at least a year at a dose of 200 mg, given 2–3 times a day [14]. Resolution of CSF abnormalities, including a negative antigen test is the recommended treatment target. Specific recommendations for CSF monitoring are: (a) worsening disease in the initial 2 weeks of therapy or lack of improvement by 1 month of therapy, in order to re-evaluate the diagnosis, (b) when amphotericin B is being replaced by a triazole, (c) if relapse is suspected and (d) after 1 year of therapy, to make the decision of treatment continuation or stoppage. Therapeutic drug monitoring for itraconazole is recommended during treatment to ensure adequate drug exposure. Treatment recommendations for histoplasmosis meningitis or CNS masses are the same. Also, for patients with concurrent pulmonary disease, chronic suppressive therapy with 200 mg of itraconazole, given once a day, is indicated until the patient's immune system is reconstituted [13, 14, 28].

The role of steroids is not well described, although case reports indicate they can be successfully used [14] . Similarly, routine brain or spinal cord surgery is not recommended by IDSA but is chronicled in case reports [14, 28]. Hydrocephalus complicating CNS histoplasmosis may be managed with shunt placement when the patient has received at least 2 weeks of amphotericin B therapy [22]. The management of increased intracranial pressure and the long-term sequelae that require rehabilitation is similar to what is done for stroke and brain tumours [14, 28].

In a sizable cohort of patients, the one-year survival of patients with CNS histoplasmosis was reported to be 75% among patients who were initially treated with liposomal or deoxycholate formulations of amphotericin [28].

3.2 Histoplasmosis in pregnancy

All presenting clinical syndromes of histoplasmosis in pregnancy require antifungal therapy due to the increased risk of trans-placental transmission of the infection to the developing fetus [29]. Preferably, pregnant women can be treated with amphotericin B preparations for 4–6 weeks. Lipid formulation of amphotericin B is given at a dose of 3–5 mg/kg/day. For pregnant women with low risk for nephrotoxicity, amphotericin B deoxycholate (0.7–1.0 mg/kg/day) may be offered as a substitute [14, 30]. Coupled with this, post-partum monitoring of the child for any evidence of the infection is vital. In any case of the newborn showing signs of histoplasmosis infection, it is recommended that treatment of amphotericin B deoxycholate (1 mg/kg/day) is given for 4 weeks [14, 30].

Itraconazole is generally considered teratogenic to the growing fetus and is therefore best avoided in pregnancy. However, itraconazole may be considered for treatment in pregnant women with systemic histoplasmosis, but only after the first trimester [31, 32]. Amphotericin B therefore remains the drug of choice in managing histoplasmosis in pregnancy, as azole antifungals should generally be avoided.

3.3 Histoplasmosis-associated immune reconstitution inflammatory syndrome in the context of human immunodeficiency virus disease

Immune reconstitution inflammatory syndrome (IRIS) is a spectrum of inflammatory disorders linked with paradoxical worsening of pre-existing infectious diseases (previously diagnosed or subclinical) in HIV-infected patients. It typically follows, the initiation of antiretroviral therapy (ART): whereby the ART improves the patient's immune system enough to mount an inflammatory response tends to unmask the underlying infectious processes, such as histoplasmosis [33–36].

In studies done among HIV patients, histoplasmosis-associated - IRIS was associated with histoplasmosis; IRIS was reported to be uncommon with incidence rates of 0.74 cases per 1000 HIV-infected person-years 0.5% [37–39]. However according to another study among 271 patients, the emergence of IRIS tended to be quite common in people with HIV and disseminated histoplasmosis; whether the IRIS is triggered by the Histoplasma or other co-infections, is still unclear [40].

For HIV patients with histoplasmosis to be considered to have histoplasmosis - associated IRIS, they should fulfil most or all of the following criteria: AIDS with low pretreatment CD4 count ($\leq$100 cells/µL), a positive immunological and virological response to ART, clinical manifestations of an inflammatory condition, association between ART initiation and appearance of clinical features of the inflammatory condition and; absence of evidence of ART resistance, patient non-compliance, drug allergy or adverse reactions, a concomitant non- fungal infection, or decreased drug levels due to malabsorption or drug-drug interactions [36, 38, 41–43].

The clinical manifestations vary from case to case, and they commonly include fever, lymphadenopathy, mucocutaneous lesions, and disseminated disease. The timeline of occurrence from initiation of ART is also varied from a few days to months, and symptoms can set in when the patient is already on the ART course or when the ART is just introduced [39, 44, 45]. Histoplasmosis-associated IRIS in HIV patients may have a predilection for females over males, with one study showing that it was four times more frequent in females than males [39].

If the symptoms of IRIS are mild, the patient is managed symptomatically. The role of steroids in treating histoplasmosis-IRIS is yet unclear [39].

However if the presentation is severe, corticosteroids may be used as they have been seen to be of benefit in TB-associated IRIS, though they should be used with caution [46].

Once a patient exhibits features of IRIS while already on effective ART, the ART should be continued and the patient should be initiated on histoplasmosis treatment immediately. However if the patient is not receiving ART, a two-week delay is encouraged before starting ART while the patient is on antifungal therapy (amphotericin B or itraconazole) as per the guidelines [14].

4. Conclusions

Itraconazole alone is used for the treatment of mild forms of histoplasmosis and as a step-down therapy in severe disease and for secondary prophylaxis to prevent relapse in the immunocompromised after induction therapy with amphotericin B. Moderate-to-severe acute pulmonary histoplasmosis as well as acute progressive disseminated histoplasmosis require intravenous amphotericin B therapy for at least 2 weeks (4–6 weeks if meningeal involvement) or until a patient can tolerate oral therapy, then oral itraconazole (or an alternative triazole) for at least 12 weeks (for acute pulmonary) or 12 months (for acute progressive disseminated histoplasmosis). Chronic cavitary pulmonary histoplasmosis is treated with itraconazole for 12–24 months. There is insufficient evidence to support the use of isavuconazole and the echinocandins for the treatment of histoplasmosis.

Author details

Felix Bongomin[1*], Richard Kwizera[2], Joseph Baruch Baluku[3,4], Lucy Grace Asio[1] and Akaninyene A. Otu[5]

1 Department of Medical Microbiology and Immunology, Faculty of Medicine, Gulu University, Gulu, Uganda

2 Translational Research Laboratory, Infectious Diseases Institute, College of Health Sciences, Makerere University, Kampala, Uganda

3 Division of Pulmonology, Mulago National Referral Hospital, Kampala, Uganda

4 Department of Programs, Mildmay Uganda, Uganda

5 Department of Internal Medicine, University of Calabar, Calabar, Nigeria

*Address all correspondence to: drbongomin@gmail.com

IntechOpen

References

[1] Daher EF, Silva GB Jr, FAS B, CFV T, RMS M, Ferreira MT, et al. Clinical and laboratory features of disseminated histoplasmosis in HIV patients from Brazil. Tropical Medicine & International Health. 2007;**12**(9):1108-1115

[2] Godwin, RA Des Prez RM. Histoplasmosis. The American Review of Respiratory Disease. 1978;**117**:929-956

[3] Garcia-Guiñon A, Torres-Rodríguez JM, Ndidongarte DT, Cortadellas F, Labrín L. Disseminated histoplasmosis by Histoplasma capsulatum var. duboisii in a paediatric patient from the Chad Republic, Africa. European Journal of Clinical Microbiology & Infectious Diseases. 2009;**28**(6):697-699

[4] Darling ST. Histoplasmosis: A fatal infectious disease resembling kala-azar found among natives of tropical America. Archives of Internal Medicine. 1908;**II**(2):107

[5] Queiroz-Telles F, Fahal AH, Falci DR, Caceres DH, Chiller T, Pasqualotto AC. Neglected endemic mycoses. The Lancet Infectious Diseases. 2017;**17**(11):e367-e377. Available from: http://www.ncbi.nlm.nih.gov/pubmed/28774696

[6] Bongomin F, Kwizera R, Denning DW. Getting histoplasmosis on the map of international recommendations for patients with advanced HIV disease. Journal of Fungi. 2019;**5**(3). Available from: http://www.ncbi.nlm.nih.gov/pubmed/31480775

[7] Nacher M, Leitao TS, Gómez BL, Couppié P, Adenis A, Damasceno L, et al. The fight against HIV-associated disseminated histoplasmosis in the Americas: Unfolding the different stories of four centers. Journal of Fungi.

2019;**5**(2). Available from: http://www.ncbi.nlm.nih.gov/pubmed/31212897

[8] Caceres DH, Valdes A. Histoplasmosis and tuberculosis co-occurrence in people with advanced HIV. Journal of Fungi. 2019;**5**(3). Available from: http://www.ncbi.nlm.nih.gov/pubmed/31404979

[9] Limper AH, Adenis A, Le T, Harrison TS. Fungal infections in HIV/AIDS. The Lancet Infectious Diseases. 2017;**17**(11):e334-e343. Available from: http://www.ncbi.nlm.nih.gov/pubmed/28774701

[10] Dylewski J. Acute pulmonary histoplasmosis. Canadian Medical Association Journal. 2011;**183**(14):E1090-E1090

[11] Inojosa W, Rossi MC, Laurino L, Giobbia M, Fuser R, Carniato A, et al. Progressive disseminated histoplasmosis among human immunodeficiency virus-infected patients from West-Africa: Report of four imported cases in Italy. Le Infezioni in Medicina. 2011;**19**(1):49-55

[12] Wheat LJ, Azar MM, Bahr NC, Spec A, Relich RF, Hage C. Histoplasmosis. Infectious Disease Clinics of North America. 2016;**30**:207-227

[13] Azar MM, Hage CA. Clinical perspectives in the diagnosis and management of histoplasmosis. Clinics in Chest Medicine. 2017;**38**(3):403-415. DOI: 10.1016/j.ccm.2017.04.004

[14] Wheat LJ, Freifeld AG, Kleiman MB, Baddley JW, McKinsey DS, Loyd JE, et al. Clinical practice guidelines for the management of patients with histoplasmosis: 2007 update by the infectious diseases society of America. Clinical Infectious Diseases. 2007;**45**(7):807-825

[15] Richardson MD, Warnock DW. Fungal Infection: Diagnosis and Mangement. 4th ed. Oxford, UK: Blackwell Publ Ltd; 2012. p. 28

[16] Nacher M, Blanchet D, Bongomin F, Chakrabarti A, Couppié P, Demar M, et al. Histoplasma capsulatum antigen detection tests as an essential diagnostic tool for patients with advanced HIV disease in low and middle income countries: A systematic review of diagnostic accuracy studies. PLoS Neglected Tropical Diseases. 2018;**12**(10):e0006802

[17] Cáceres DH, Samayoa BE, Medina NG, Tobón AM, Guzmán BJ, Mercado D, et al. Multicenter validation of commercial antigenuria reagents to diagnose progressive disseminated histoplasmosis in people living with HIV/AIDS in two Latin American countries. The Journal of Clinical Microbiology. 2018;**56**(6):e01959-17. Available from: http://jcm.asm.org/lookup/doi/10.1128/JCM.01959-17

[18] Bellmann R, Smuszkiewicz P. Pharmacokinetics of antifungal drugs: Practical implications for optimized treatment of patients. Infection. 2017;**45**(6):737-779. DOI: 10.1007/s15010-017-1042-z

[19] Campoy S, Adrio JL. Antifungals. Biochemical Pharmacology. 2017;**133**: 86-96. Available from: https://linkinghub.elsevier.com/retrieve/pii/S0006295216304221

[20] Kauffman CA. Histoplasmosis. Clinics in Chest Medicine. 2009;**30**(2):217-225

[21] Joint Formulary Committee. British national formulary. The BMJ. 2020:79. Available from: http://www.ncbi.nlm.nih.gov/pubmed/10981569

[22] Wheat LJ, Musial CE, Jenny-Avital E. Diagnosis and management of central nervous system histoplasmosis. Clinical Infectious Diseases. 2005;**40**(6):844-852

[23] Haynes RR, Connolly PA, Durkin MM, AM LM, Smedema ML, Brizendine E, et al. Antifungal therapy for central nervous system Histoplasmosis, using a newly developed intracranial model of infection. The Journal of Infectious Diseases. 2002;**185**(12):1830-1832

[24] Ramireddy S, Wanger A, Ostrosky L. An instructive case of CNS histoplasmosis in an immunocompetent host. Medical Mycology Case Reports. 2012;**1**(1):69-71

[25] Prinapori R, Mikulska M, Parisini A, Ratto S, Viscoli C. A case of cerebral histoplasmosis in an immunocompetent host successfully treated with voriconazole. Infectious Diseases & Tropical Medicine. 2015;**1**(2):1-4

[26] Eid AJ, Leever JD, Husmann K. Compartmentalized Histoplasma capsulatum infection of the central nervous system. Case Reports in Infectious Diseases. 2015;**2015**:1-3. Available from: http://www.hindawi.com/journals/criid/2015/581415/

[27] Schestatsky P, Chedid MF, Amaral OB, Unis G, Oliveira FM, Severo LC. Isolated central nervous system histoplasmosis in immunocompetent hosts: A series of 11 cases. Scandinavian Journal of Infectious Diseases. 2006;**38**(1):43-48. Available from: http://www.tandfonline.com/doi/full/10.1080/00365540500372895

[28] Wheat J, Myint T, Guo Y, Kemmer P, Hage C, Terry C, et al. Central nervous system histoplasmosis. Medicine. 2018;**97**(13):1-8

[29] Whitt SP, Koch GA, Fender B, Ratnasamy N, Everett ED. Histoplasmosis in pregnancy: Case series and report of transplacental

transmission. Archives of Internal Medicine. 2004;**164**(4):454-458

[30] Moudgal VV, Sobel JD. Antifungal drugs in pregnancy: A review. Expert Opinion on Drug Safety. 2003;**2**(5):475-483

[31] De Santis M, Di Gianantonio E, Cesari E, Ambrosini G, Straface G, Clementi M. First-trimester itraconazole exposure and pregnancy outcome: A prospective cohort study of women contacting teratology information services in Italy. Drug Safety. 2009;**32**(3):239-244

[32] Bar-Oz B, Moretti ME, Bishai R, Mareels G, Van Tittelboom T, Verspeelt J, et al. Pregnancy outcome after in utero exposure to itraconazole: A prospective cohort study. American Journal of Obstetrics and Gynecology. 2000;**183**(3):617-620

[33] Michelet C, Arvieux C, Francois C, Besnier JM, Rogez JP, Breux JP, et al. Opportunistic infections occurring during highly active antiretroviral treatment. AIDS. 1998;**12**(14):1815-1822

[34] Hirsch HH, Kaufmann G, Sendi P, Battegay M. Immune reconstitution in HIV-infected patients. Clinical Infectious Diseases. 2004;**38**(8):1159-1166

[35] French MA, Lenzo N, John M, Mallal SA, McKinnon EJ, James IR, et al. Immune restoration disease after the treatment of immunodeficient HIV-infected patients with highly active antiretroviral therapy. HIV Medicine. 2000;**1**(2):107-115

[36] Shelburne SA, Montes M, Hamill RJ. Immune reconstitution inflammatory syndrome: More answers, more questions. The Journal of Antimicrobial Chemotherapy. 2006;**57**(2):167-170

[37] Couppie P, Aznar C, Carme B, Nacher M. American histoplasmosis in developing countries with a special focus on patients with HIV: Diagnosis, treatment, and prognosis. Current Opinion in Infectious Diseases. 2006;**19**(5):443-449

[38] Novak RM, Richardson JT, Buchacz K, Chmiel JS, Durham MD, Palella FJ, et al. Immune reconstitution inflammatory syndrome: Incidence and implications for mortality. AIDS. 2012;**26**(6):721-730

[39] Melzani A, de Reynal de Saint MR, Ntab B, Djossou F, Epelboin L, Nacher M, et al. Incidence and trends in immune reconstitution inflammatory syndrome associated with histoplasma capsulatum among people living with human immunodeficiency virus: A 20-year case series and literature review. Clinical Infectious Diseases. 2020;**70**(4):643-652

[40] Boulougoura A, Laidlaw E, Roby G, Mejia Y, Pau A, Sheikh V, et al. Immune reconstitution inflammatory syndrome in patients with HIV/AIDS and Histoplasmosis: A case series. Open Forum Infectious Diseases. 2019;**6**(Supplement_2):S195-S195

[41] Ratnam I, Chiu C, Kandala N-B, Easterbrook PJ. Incidence and risk factors for immune reconstitution inflammatory syndrome in an ethnically diverse HIV type 1-infected cohort. Clinical Infectious Diseases. 2006;**42**(3):418-427

[42] Breton G, Duval X, Estellat C, Poaletti X, Bonnet D, Mvondo Mvondo D, et al. Determinants of immune reconstitution inflammatory syndrome in HIV type 1-infected patients with tuberculosis after initiation of antiretroviral therapy. Clinical Infectious Diseases. 2004;**39**(11):1709-1712

[43] Manabe YC, Campbell JD, Sydnor E, Moore RD. Immune reconstitution inflammatory syndrome:

Risk factors and treatment implications. Journal of Acquired Immune Deficiency Syndromes. 2007;**46**(4):456-462

[44] Kiggundu R, Nabeta HW, Okia R, Rhein J, Lukande R. Unmasking histoplasmosis immune reconstitution inflammatory syndrome in a patient recently started on antiretroviral therapy. Autopsy & Case Reports. 2016;**6**(4):27-33

[45] Passos L, Talhari C, Santos M, Ribeiro-Rodrigues R, Ferreira LC de L, Talhari S. Histoplasmosis-associated immune reconstitution inflammatory syndrome. Anais Brasileiros de Dermatologia. 2011;**86**(4 Suppl 1): S168-S172

[46] Meintjes G, Scriven J, Marais S. Management of the immune reconstitution inflammatory syndrome. Current HIV/AIDS Reports. 2012;**9**(3):238-250